# FAVORITE BRAND NAME

# DIABETIC RECIPES

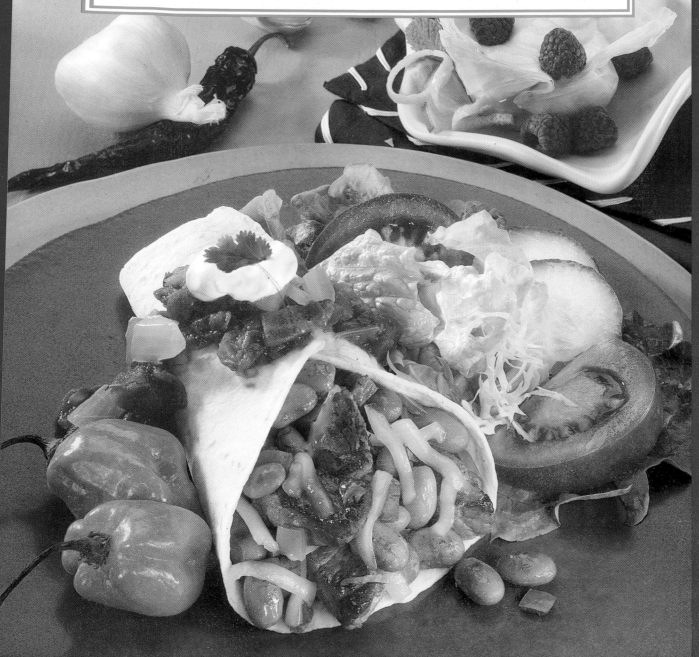

# FAVORITE BRAND NAME

# DIABETIC RECIPES

# Appetizers & Snacks

## Vegetable-Topped Hummus

*Look for tahini, a thick paste made from ground sesame seeds, in Middle Eastern markets, health food stores or the ethnic section of large supermarkets.*

**1 can (about 15 ounces) chick-peas, rinsed and drained**
**2 tablespoons tahini**
**2 tablespoons lemon juice**
**1 clove garlic**
**¾ teaspoon salt**
**1 tomato, finely chopped**
**2 green onions, finely chopped**
**2 tablespoons chopped parsley**

1. Combine chick-peas, tahini, lemon juice, garlic and salt in food processor; process until smooth.

2. Combine tomato, green onions and parsley in small bowl.

3. Place chick-pea mixture in medium serving bowl; spoon tomato mixture evenly over top. Serve with wedges of pita bread or assorted crackers.

*Makes 8 servings*

**Nutrients per Serving:** Calories: 82 (31% Calories from Fat), Total Fat: 3 g,
Saturated Fat: trace, Protein: 3 g, Carbohydrate: 11 g, Cholesterol: 0 mg,
Sodium: 429 mg, Fiber: 3 g, Sugar: 1 g
**Dietary Exchanges:** ½ Starch/Bread, 1 Vegetable, ½ Fat

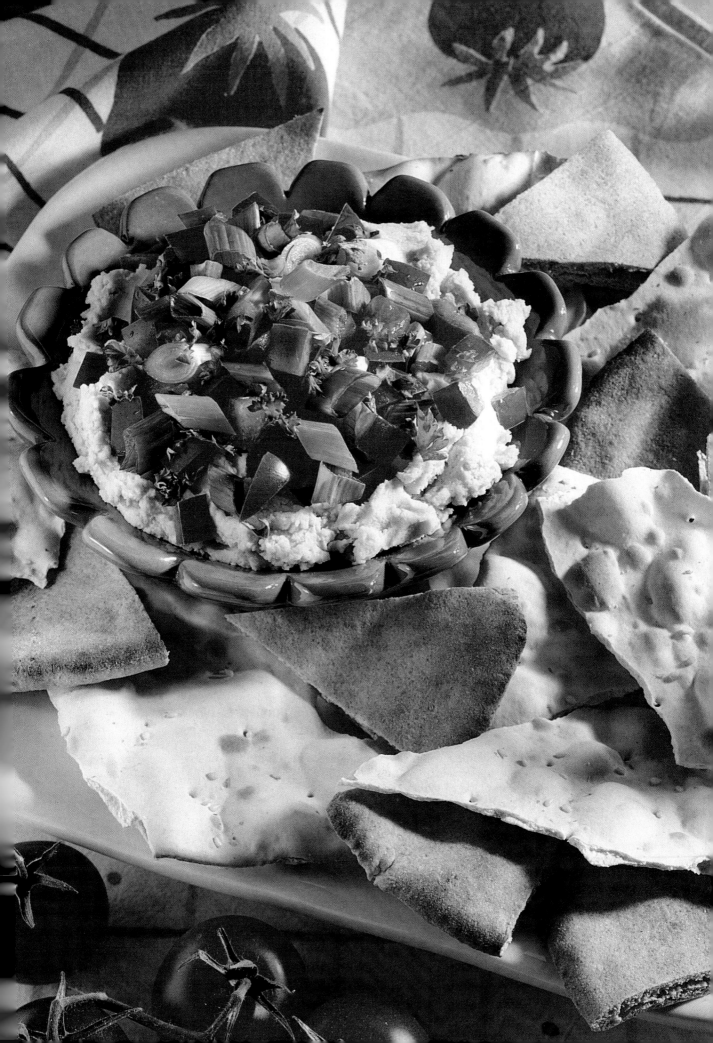

# Cinnamon Caramel Corn

**8 cups air-popped popcorn (about ⅓ cup kernels)**
**2 tablespoons honey**
**4 teaspoons margarine**
**¼ teaspoon ground cinnamon**

1. Preheat oven to 350°F. Spray jelly-roll pan with nonstick cooking spray. Place popcorn in large bowl.

2. Stir honey, margarine and cinnamon in small saucepan over low heat until margarine is melted and mixture is smooth; immediately pour over popcorn. Toss with spoon to coat evenly. Pour onto prepared pan; bake 12 to 14 minutes or until coating is golden brown and appears crackled, stirring twice. Let cool on pan 5 minutes. (As popcorn cools, coating becomes crisp. If not crisp enough, or if popcorn softens upon standing, return to oven and heat 5 to 8 minutes more.)            *Makes 4 servings*

**Nutrients per Serving:** Calories: 117 (29% Calories from Fat), Total Fat: 4 g, Saturated Fat: 1 g, Protein: 2 g, Carbohydrate: 19 g, Cholesterol: 0 mg, Sodium: 45 mg, Fiber: 1 g, Sugar: 9 g
**Dietary Exchanges:** 1 Starch/Bread, 1 Fat

## Variations

*Cajun Popcorn:* Preheat oven and prepare jelly-roll pan as directed above. Combine 7 teaspoons honey, 4 teaspoons margarine and 1 teaspoon Cajun or Creole seasoning in small saucepan. Proceed with recipe as directed above. Makes 4 servings.

**Nutrients per Serving:** Calories: 122 (28% Calories from Fat), Total Fat: 4 g, Saturated Fat: 1 g, Protein: 2 g, Carbohydrate: 20 g, Cholesterol: 0 mg, Sodium: 91 mg, Fiber: 1 g, Sugar: 10 g
**Dietary Exchanges:** 1½ Starch/Bread, ½ Fat

*Italian Popcorn:* Spray 8 cups of air-popped popcorn with fat-free butter-flavored spray to coat. Sprinkle with 2 tablespoons finely grated Parmesan cheese, ⅛ teaspoon black pepper and ½ teaspoon dried oregano leaves. Gently toss to coat. Makes 4 servings.

**Nutrients per Serving:** Calories: 65 (14% Calories from Fat), Total Fat: 1 g, Saturated Fat: 1 g, Protein: 3 g, Carbohydrate: 10 g, Cholesterol: 2 mg, Sodium: 58 mg, Fiber: 1 g, Sugar: 0 g
**Dietary Exchanges:** 1 Starch/Bread

*Clockwise from top: Italian Popcorn, Cinnamon Caramel Corn and Cajun Popcorn*

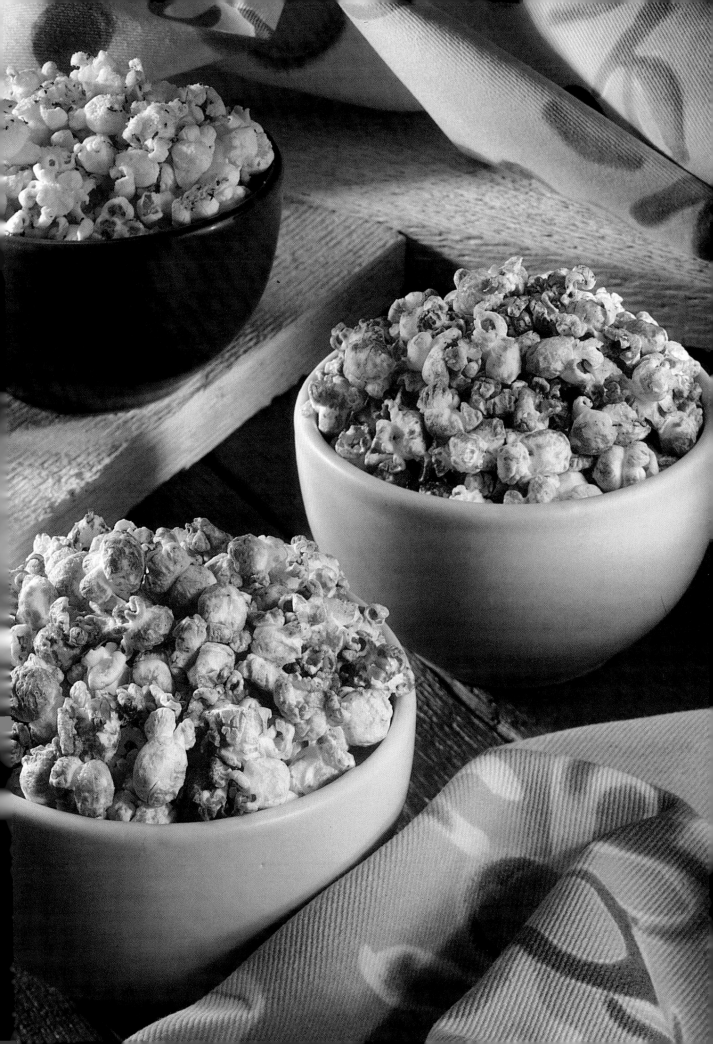

# Greek Spinach-Cheese Rolls

*Keep these savory rolls on hand for a quick pick-me-up or serve along side soup or salad.*

**1 loaf (1 pound) frozen bread dough**
**1 package (10 ounces) frozen chopped spinach, thawed and**
    **squeezed dry**
**¾ cup (3 ounces) crumbled feta cheese**
**½ cup (2 ounces) shredded reduced-fat Monterey Jack cheese**
**4 green onions, thinly sliced**
**1 teaspoon dried dill weed**
**½ teaspoon garlic powder**
**½ teaspoon black pepper**

1. Thaw bread dough according to package directions. Spray 15 muffin cups with nonstick cooking spray; set aside. Roll out dough on lightly floured surface to 15×9-inch rectangle. (If dough is springy and difficult to roll, cover with plastic wrap and let rest 5 minutes to relax.) Position dough so long edge runs parallel to edge of work surface.

2. Combine spinach, cheeses, green onions, dill weed, garlic powder and pepper in large bowl; mix well.

3. Sprinkle spinach mixture evenly over dough to within 1 inch of long edges. Starting at long edge, roll up snugly, pinching seam closed. Place seam side down; cut roll with serrated knife into 1-inch-wide slices. Place slices cut sides up in prepared muffin cups. Cover with plastic wrap; let stand 30 minutes in warm place until rolls are slightly puffy.

4. Preheat oven to 375°F. Bake 20 to 25 minutes or until golden. Serve warm or at room temperature. Rolls can be stored in refrigerator in airtight container up to 2 days.              *Makes 15 servings (1 roll each)*

**Nutrients per Serving:** Calories: 111 (24% Calories from Fat), Total Fat: 3 g,
Saturated Fat: 2 g, Protein: 5 g, Carbohydrate: 16 g, Cholesterol: 8 mg,
Sodium: 267 mg, Fiber: trace, Sugar: trace
**Dietary Exchanges:** 1 Starch/Bread, ½ Lean Meat, ½ Fat

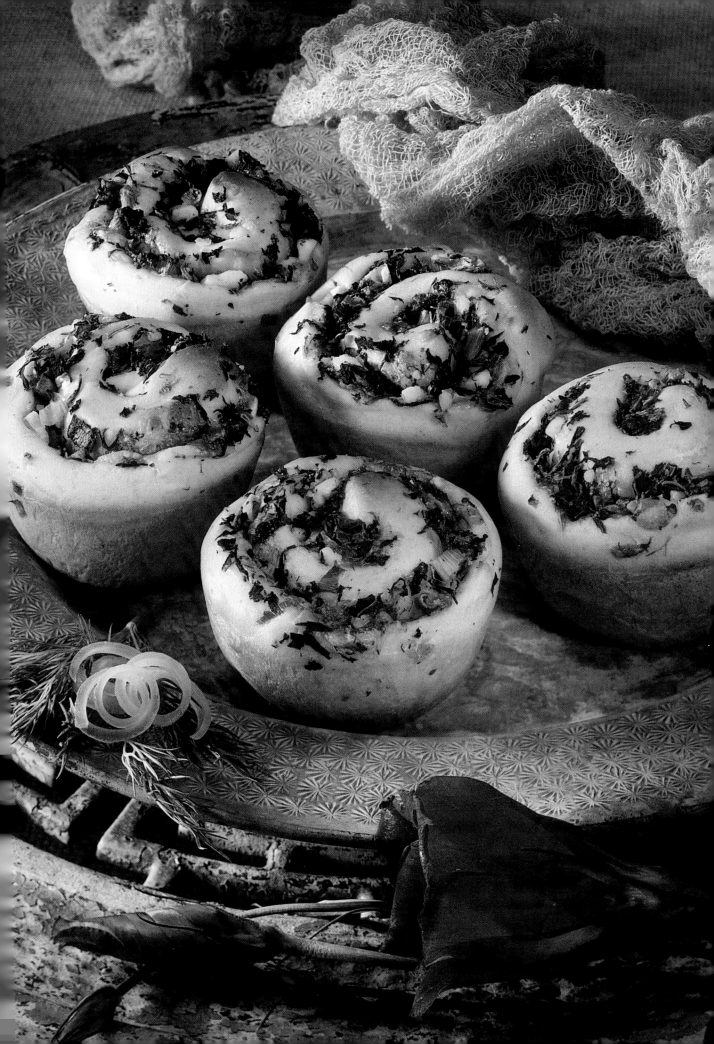

# Venezuelan Salsa

*Try a taste-tempting tropical sensation! This unusual salsa makes a terrific appetizer, or serve it with fruit salads, grilled chicken or fish.*

   **1 mango, peeled, pitted and diced**
  **½ medium papaya, peeled, seeded and diced**
  **½ medium avocado, peeled, pitted and diced**
   **1 carrot, finely chopped**
   **1 small onion, finely chopped**
   **1 rib celery, finely chopped**
     **Juice of 1 lemon**
   **3 cloves garlic, minced**
   **2 tablespoons chopped cilantro**
   **1 jalapeño pepper,\* finely chopped**
 **1½ teaspoons ground cumin**
  **½ teaspoon salt**

\*Jalapeño peppers can sting and irritate the skin; wear rubber gloves when handling peppers and do not touch eyes. Wash hands after handling.

1. Combine all ingredients in medium bowl. Refrigerate several hours to allow flavors to blend. Serve with baked tortilla chips, carrot and celery sticks or apple wedges.            *Makes 10 servings (¼ cup each)*

**Nutrients per Serving:** Calories: 52 (27% Calories from Fat), Total Fat: 2 g, Saturated Fat: trace, Protein: 1 g, Carbohydrate: 9 g, Cholesterol: 0 mg, Sodium: 117 mg, Fiber: 2 g, Sugar: 5 g
**Dietary Exchanges:** 1 Fruit

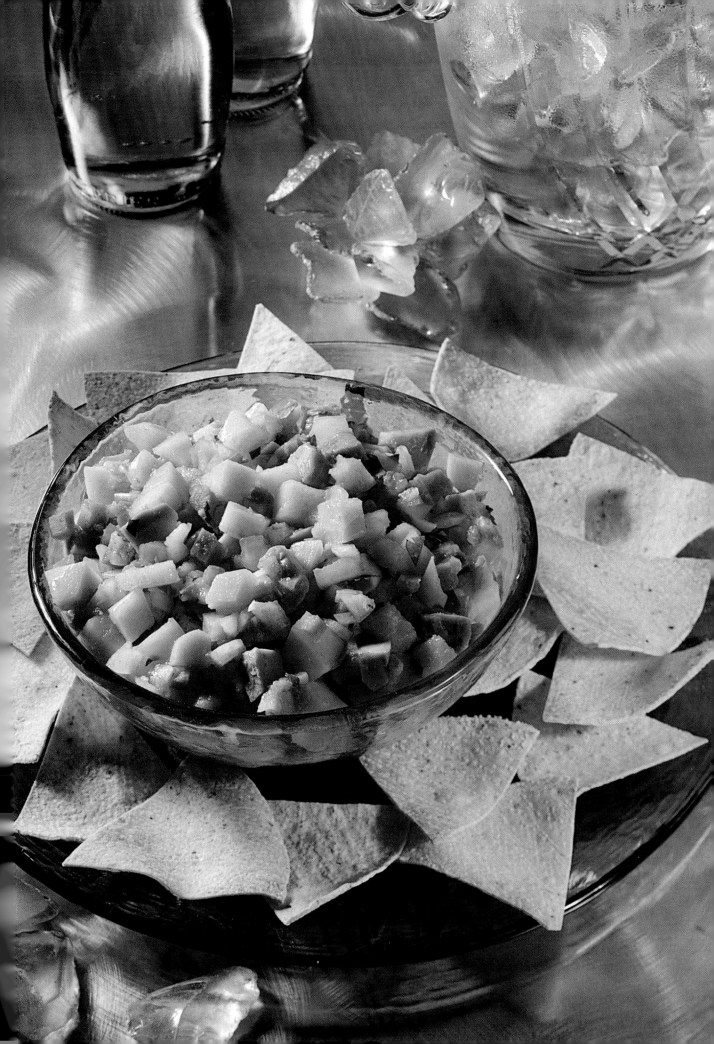

# Banana & Chocolate Chip Pops

*Three-ounce paper cups can be used in place of popsicle molds. Spoon yogurt mixture into paper cups, insert wooden stick in center of each and freeze. To prevent popsicles from tipping over, simply stand cups in a muffin pan after filling. To unmold, peel paper cup away.*

**1 small ripe banana**
**1 carton (8 ounces) banana nonfat yogurt**
**⅛ teaspoon ground nutmeg**
**2 tablespoons mini chocolate chips**

1. Slice banana; place in food processor with yogurt and nutmeg. Process until smooth. Transfer to small bowl; stir in chips.

2. Spoon banana mixture into 4 plastic popsicle molds. Place tops on molds; set in provided stand. Set on level surface in freezer; freeze 2 hours or until firm. To unmold, briefly run warm water over popsicle molds until each pop loosens. *Makes 4 servings*

**Nutrients per Serving:** Calories: 103 (14% Calories from Fat), Total Fat: 2 g, Saturated Fat: trace, Protein: 3 g, Carbohydrate: 20 g, Cholesterol: 1 mg, Sodium: 37 mg, Fiber: trace, Sugar: 16 g
**Dietary Exchanges:** 1½ Fruit

## Variations

**Peanut Butter & Jelly Pops:** Stir ¼ cup reduced-fat peanut butter in small bowl until smooth; stir in 1 carton (8 ounces) vanilla nonfat yogurt. Drop 2 tablespoons all-fruit strawberry preserves on top of mixture; pull spoon back and forth through mixture several times to swirl slightly. Spoon into 4 molds and freeze as directed above. Makes 4 servings.

**Nutrients per Serving:** Calories: 169 (32% Calories from Fat), Total Fat: 6 g, Saturated Fat: 1 g, Protein: 7 g, Carbohydrate: 21 g, Cholesterol: 0 mg, Sodium: 131 mg, Fiber: 1 g, Sugar: 1 g
**Dietary Exchanges:** 1½ Starch/Bread, ½ Lean Meat, 1 Fat

**Blueberry-Lime Pops:** Stir 1 carton (8 ounces) Key lime nonfat yogurt in small bowl until smooth; fold in ⅓ cup frozen blueberries. Spoon into 4 molds and freeze as directed above. Makes 4 servings.

**Nutrients per Serving:** Calories: 57 (1% Calories from Fat), Total Fat: trace, Saturated Fat: trace, Protein: 2 g, Carbohydrate: 12 g, Cholesterol: 0 mg, Sodium: 32 mg, Fiber: trace, Sugar: 10 g
**Dietary Exchanges:** 1 Fruit

*Clockwise from top: Peanut Butter & Jelly Pop, Blueberry-Lime Pop and Banana & Chocolate Chip Pop*

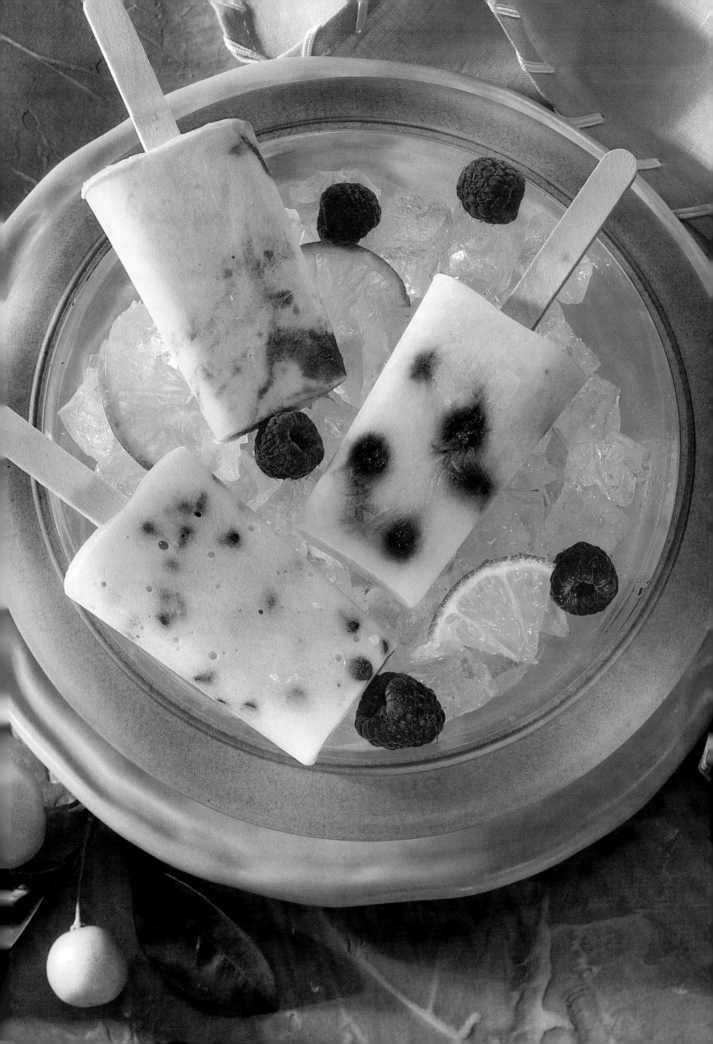

# Tuscan White Bean Crostini

*For a refreshing light lunch, serve the white bean mixture as a salad on a bed of Bibb lettuce leaves.*

**2 cans (15 ounces each) white beans (such as Great Northern or cannellini), rinsed and drained**
**½ large red bell pepper, finely chopped *or* ⅓ cup finely chopped roasted red bell pepper**
**⅓ cup finely chopped onion**
**⅓ cup red wine vinegar**
**3 tablespoons chopped parsley**
**1 tablespoon olive oil**
**2 cloves garlic, minced**
**½ teaspoon dried oregano leaves**
**¼ teaspoon black pepper**
**18 French bread slices, about ¼ inch thick**

1. Combine beans, bell pepper and onion in large bowl.

2. Whisk together vinegar, parsley, oil, garlic, oregano and black pepper in small bowl. Pour over bean mixture; toss to coat. Cover; refrigerate 2 hours or overnight.

3. Arrange bread slices in single layer on large nonstick baking sheet or broiler pan. Broil, 6 to 8 inches from heat, 30 to 45 seconds or until bread slices are lightly toasted. Remove; cool completely.

4. Top each toasted bread slice with about 3 tablespoons of bean mixture.

*Makes 6 servings*

**Nutrients per Serving:** Calories: 317 (12% Calories from Fat), Total Fat: 4 g, Saturated Fat: 1 g, Protein: 15 g, Carbohydrate: 57 g, Cholesterol: 0 mg, Sodium: 800 mg, Fiber: 1 g, Sugar: trace
**Dietary Exchanges:** 2 Starch/Bread, 1 Vegetable, ½ Fat

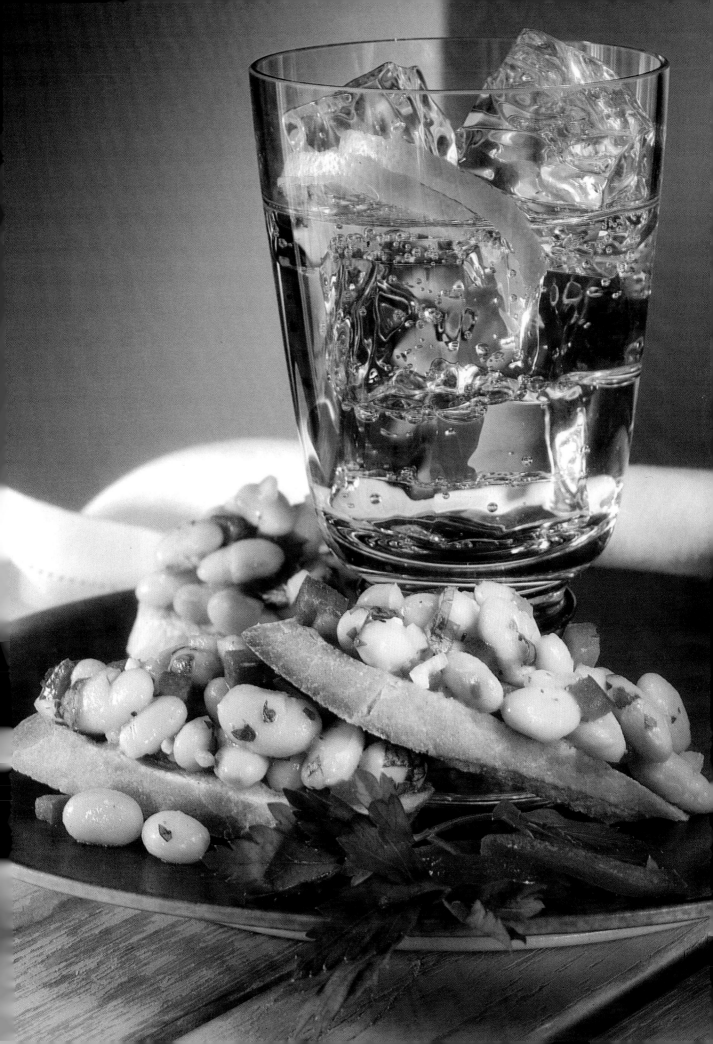

# Apricot-Chicken Pot Stickers

    2 cups plus 1 tablespoon water, divided
    2 small boneless skinless chicken breasts (about 8 ounces)
    2 cups chopped finely shredded cabbage
    ½ cup all-fruit apricot preserves
    2 green onions with tops, finely chopped
    2 teaspoons soy sauce
    ½ teaspoon grated fresh ginger
    ⅛ teaspoon black pepper
    30 (3-inch) wonton wrappers
       Prepared sweet & sour sauce (optional)

1. Bring 2 cups water to boil in medium saucepan. Add chicken. Reduce heat to low; simmer, covered, 10 minutes or until chicken is no longer pink in center. Remove from saucepan; drain.

2. Add cabbage and remaining 1 tablespoon water to saucepan. Cook over high heat 1 to 2 minutes or until water evaporates, stirring occasionally. Remove from heat; cool slightly.

3. Finely chop chicken. Add to saucepan along with preserves, green onions, soy sauce, ginger and pepper; mix well.

4. To assemble pot stickers, remove 3 wonton wrappers at a time from package. Spoon slightly rounded tablespoonful of chicken mixture onto center of each wrapper; brush edges with water. Bring 4 corners together; press to seal. Repeat with remaining wrappers and filling.

5. Spray steamer with nonstick cooking spray. Assemble steamer so that water is ½ inch below steamer basket. Fill steamer basket with pot stickers, leaving enough space between them to prevent sticking. Cover; steam 5 minutes. Transfer pot stickers to serving plate. Serve with prepared sweet & sour sauce, if desired.          *Makes 10 servings (3 pot stickers each)*

**Nutrients per Serving:** Calories: 145 (6% Calories from Fat), Total Fat: 1 g, Saturated Fat: trace, Protein: 8 g, Carbohydrate: 26 g, Cholesterol: 17 mg, Sodium: 223 mg, Fiber: 1 g, Sugar: 10 g
**Dietary Exchanges:** 1½ Starch/Bread, ½ Lean Meat

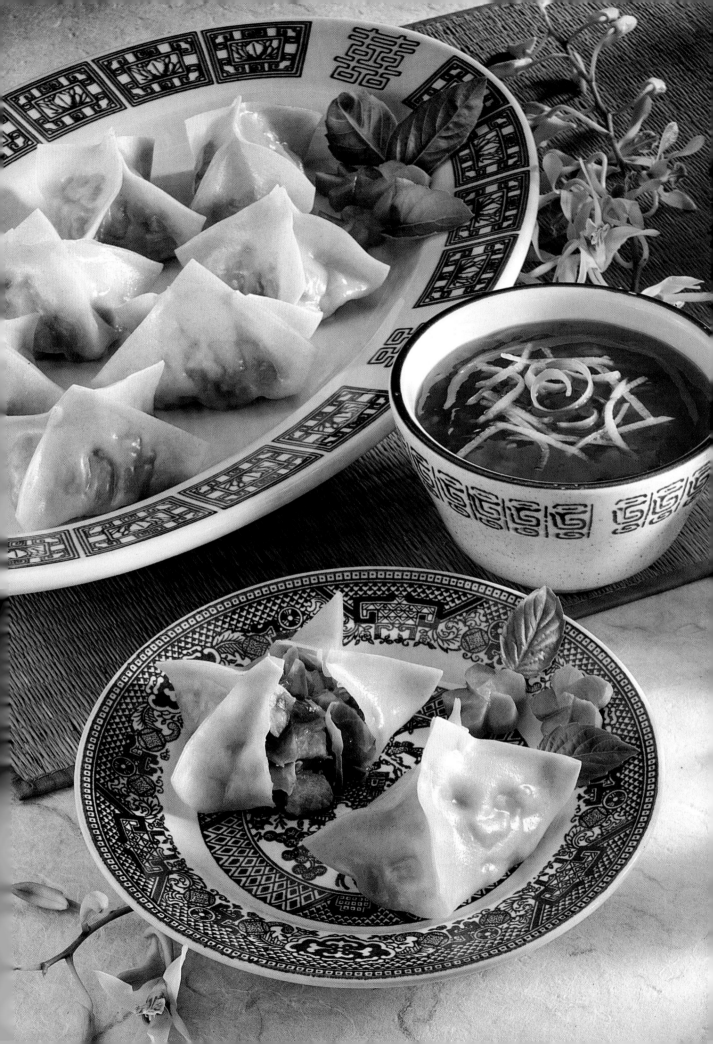

# Soups & Salads

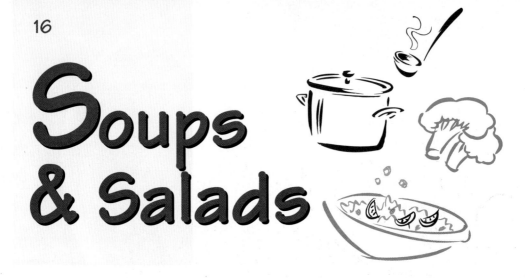

## Italian Crouton Salad

6 ounces French or Italian bread
¼ cup plain nonfat yogurt
¼ cup red wine vinegar
4 teaspoons olive oil
1 tablespoon water
3 cloves garlic, minced
6 medium (about 12 ounces) plum tomatoes
½ medium red onion, thinly sliced
3 tablespoons slivered fresh basil leaves
2 tablespoons finely chopped parsley
12 leaves red leaf lettuce *or* 4 cups prepared Italian salad mix
2 tablespoons grated Parmesan cheese

1. Preheat broiler. Cut bread into ¾-inch cubes. Place in single layer on jelly-roll pan. Broil, 4 inches from heat, 3 minutes or until bread is golden, stirring every 30 seconds to 1 minute. Remove from baking sheet; place in large bowl.

2. Whisk together yogurt, vinegar, oil, water and garlic in small bowl until blended; set aside. Core tomatoes; cut into ¼-inch-wide slices. Add to bread along with onion, basil and parsley; stir until blended. Pour yogurt mixture over crouton mixture; toss to coat. Cover; refrigerate 30 minutes or up to 1 day. (Croutons will be more tender the following day.)

3. To serve, place lettuce on plates. Spoon crouton mixture over lettuce. Sprinkle with Parmesan cheese. *Makes 6 servings*

**Nutrients per Serving:** Calories: 160 (28% Calories from Fat), Total Fat: 5 g, Saturated Fat: 1 g, Protein: 6 g, Carbohydrate: 25 g, Cholesterol: 2 mg, Sodium: 234 mg, Fiber: 2 g, Sugar: 5 g
**Dietary Exchanges:** 1 Starch/Bread, 1½ Vegetable, 1 Fat

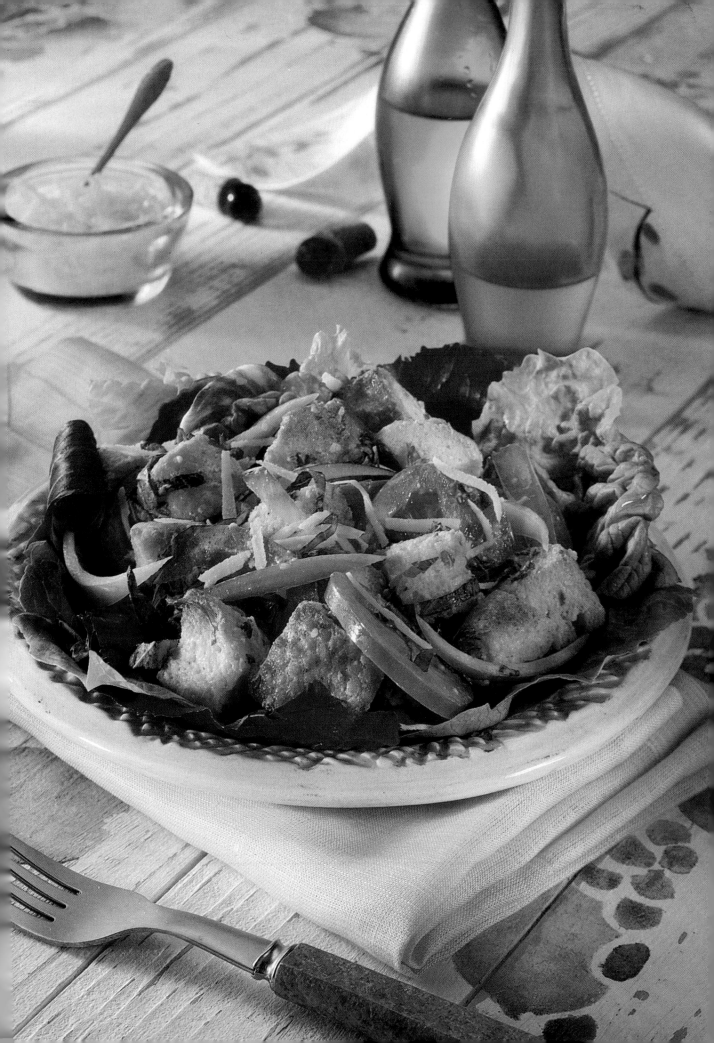

# Indian Carrot Soup

*Vitamin-rich and inexpensive, carrots star in this rich and spicy soup without the addition of any cream. This soup can be made with winter squash, such as butternut, acorn or hubbard, in place of the carrots.*

> **Nonstick cooking spray**
> **1 small onion, chopped**
> **1 tablespoon minced fresh ginger**
> **1 teaspoon olive oil**
> **1½ teaspoons curry powder**
> **½ teaspoon ground cumin**
> **2 cans (about 14 ounces each) fat-free reduced-sodium chicken broth, divided**
> **1 pound peeled baby carrots**
> **1 tablespoon sugar**
> **¼ teaspoon ground cinnamon**
> **Pinch ground red pepper**
> **2 teaspoons fresh lime juice**
> **3 tablespoons chopped cilantro**
> **¼ cup plain nonfat yogurt**

1. Spray large saucepan with cooking spray; heat over medium heat. Add onion and ginger; reduce heat to low. Cover; cook 3 to 4 minutes or until onion is transparent and crisp-tender, stirring occasionally. Add olive oil; cook and stir, uncovered, 3 to 4 minutes or until onion just turns golden. Add curry powder and cumin; cook and stir 30 seconds or until fragrant. Add 1 can chicken broth and carrots; bring to a boil over high heat. Reduce heat to low; simmer, covered, 15 minutes or until carrots are tender.

2. Ladle carrot mixture into food processor; process until smooth. Return to saucepan; stir in remaining 1 can chicken broth, sugar, cinnamon and red pepper; bring to a boil over medium heat. Remove from heat; stir in lime juice. Ladle into bowls; sprinkle with cilantro. Top each serving with 1 tablespoon yogurt.                                    *Makes 4 servings*

**Nutrients per Serving:** Calories: 99 (20% Calories from Fat), Total Fat: 2 g, Saturated Fat: trace, Protein: 3 g, Carbohydrate: 17 g, Cholesterol: trace, Sodium: 77 mg, Fiber: 1 g, Sugar: 4 g
**Dietary Exchanges:** ½ Starch/Bread, 3 Vegetable, 1 Fat

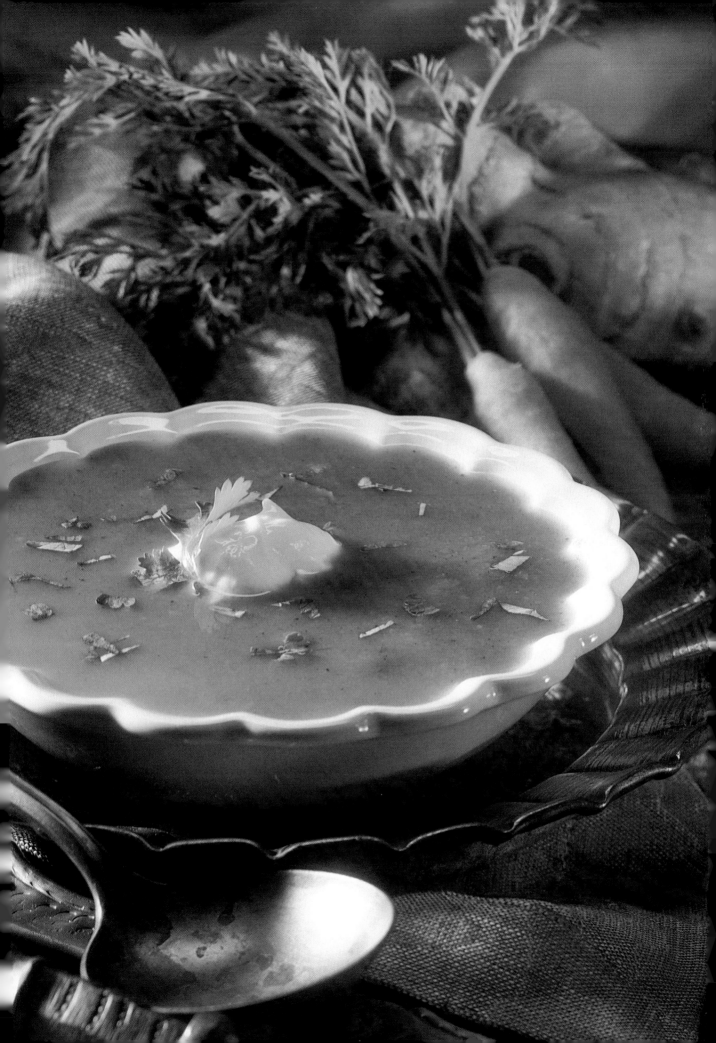

# Caribbean Cole Slaw

*Mangoes add a tropical twist to this familiar salad and provide plenty of vitamins A and C.*

**Orange-Mango Dressing (recipe follows)**
**8 cups shredded green cabbage**
**1½ large mangoes, peeled, pitted and diced**
**½ medium red bell pepper, thinly sliced**
**½ medium yellow bell pepper, thinly sliced**
**6 green onions, thinly sliced**
**¼ cup chopped cilantro**

1. Prepare Orange-Mango Dressing.

2. Combine cabbage, mangoes, bell peppers, green onions and cilantro in large bowl; stir gently to mix evenly. Pour in Orange-Mango Dressing; toss gently to coat. Serve, or store in refrigerator up to 1 day.

*Makes 6 servings*

## Orange-Mango Dressing

**½ mango, peeled, pitted and cubed**
**1 carton (6 ounces) plain nonfat yogurt**
**¼ cup frozen orange juice concentrate**
**3 tablespoons fresh lime juice**
**½ to 1 jalapeño pepper,* stemmed, seeded and minced**
**1 teaspoon finely minced fresh ginger**

*Jalapeño peppers can sting and irritate the skin; wear rubber gloves when handling peppers and do not touch eyes. Wash hands after handling.

1. Place mango in food processor; process until smooth. Add remaining ingredients; process until smooth.

*Makes about 1 cup*

**Nutrients per Serving:** Calories: 124 (4% Calories from Fat), Total Fat: 1 g, Saturated Fat: trace, Protein: 4 g, Carbohydrate: 28 g, Cholesterol: 1 mg, Sodium: 52 mg, Fiber: 4 g, Sugar: 16 g
**Dietary Exchanges:** 2 Fruit

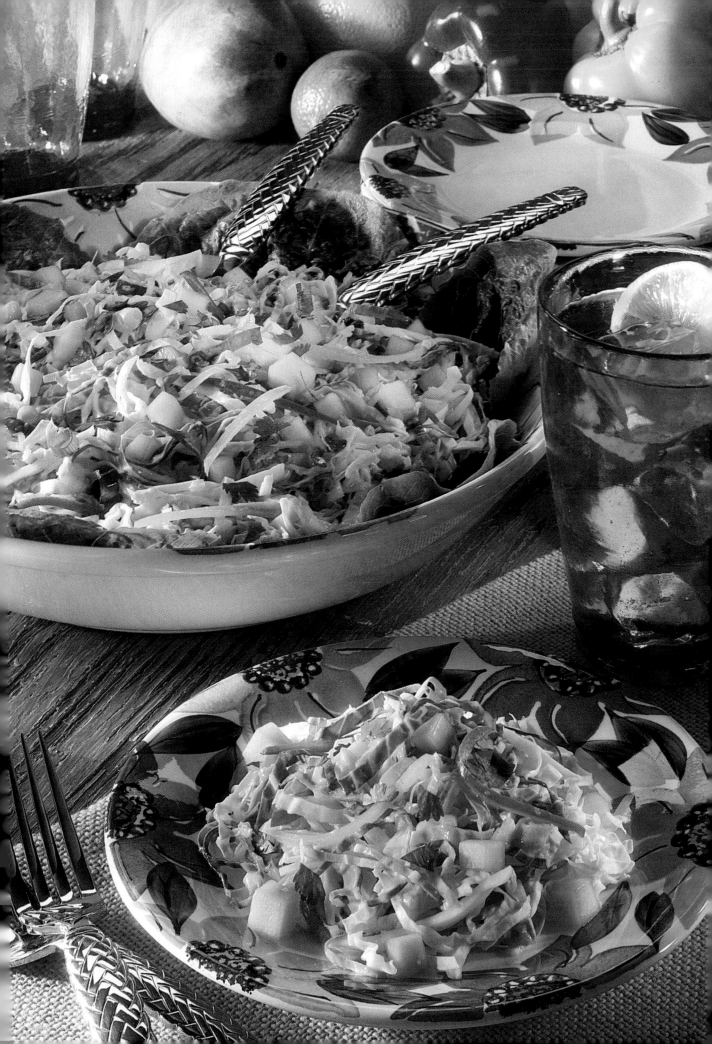

# Southwest Corn and Turkey Soup

*Dry chilies add a rich earthy flavor not achievable with their fresh counterparts.*

**3 dried ancho chilies (each about 4 inches long) *or* 6 dried New
  Mexico chilies (each about 6 inches long)**
**2 small zucchini**
  **Nonstick cooking spray**
**1 medium onion, thinly sliced**
**3 cloves garlic, minced**
**1 teaspoon ground cumin**
**3 cans (about 14 ounces each) fat-free reduced-sodium chicken broth**
**1½ to 2 cups (8 to 12 ounces) shredded cooked dark turkey meat**
**1 can (15 ounces) chick-peas or black beans, rinsed and drained**
**1 package (10 ounces) frozen corn**
**¼ cup cornmeal**
**1 teaspoon dried oregano leaves**
**⅓ cup chopped cilantro**

1. Cut stems from chilies; shake out seeds. Place chilies in medium bowl; cover with boiling water. Let stand 20 to 40 minutes or until chilies are soft; drain. Cut open lengthwise and lay flat on work surface. With edge of small knife, scrape chili pulp from skin (thicker-skinned ancho chilies will yield more flesh than thinner-skinned New Mexico chilies). Finely mince pulp; set aside.

2. Cut zucchini in half lengthwise; slice crosswise into ½-inch-wide pieces. Set aside.

3. Spray large saucepan with cooking spray; heat over medium heat. Add onion; cook, covered, 3 to 4 minutes or until light golden brown, stirring several times. Add garlic and cumin; cook and stir about 30 seconds or until fragrant. Add chicken broth, reserved chili pulp, zucchini, turkey, chick-peas, corn, cornmeal and oregano; bring to a boil over high heat. Reduce heat to low; simmer 15 minutes or until zucchini is tender. Stir in cilantro; ladle into bowls and serve.                    *Makes 6 servings*

**Nutrients per Serving:** Calories: 243 (19% Calories from Fat), Total Fat: 5 g,
Saturated Fat: 1 g, Protein: 19 g, Carbohydrate: 32 g, Cholesterol: 32 mg,
Sodium: 408 mg, Fiber: 7 g, Sugar: 2 g
**Dietary Exchanges:** 2 Bread/Starch, 2 Lean Meat

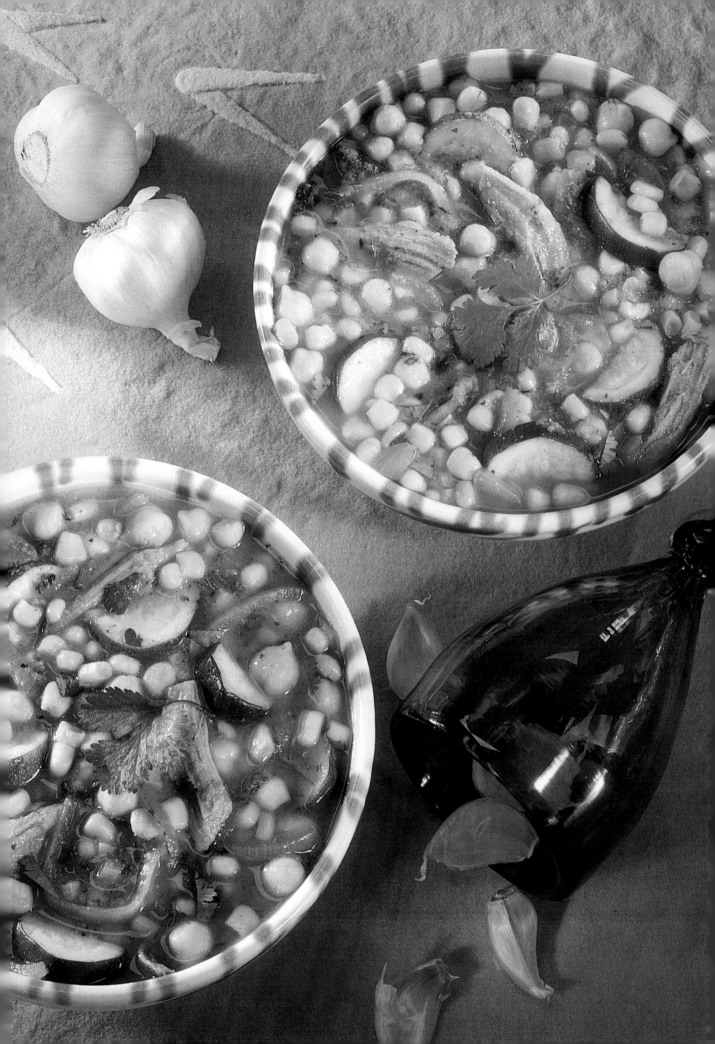

# Scallop and Spinach Salad

*The combination of scallops, blue cheese and toasted walnuts turn the familiar spinach salad into a delicious new creation.*

   1 package (10 ounces) spinach leaves, washed, stemmed and torn
   3 thin slices red onion, halved and separated
  12 ounces sea scallops
     Ground red pepper
     Paprika
     Nonstick cooking spray
  ½ cup prepared fat-free Italian salad dressing
  ¼ cup crumbled blue cheese
   2 tablespoons toasted walnuts

1. Pat spinach dry; place in large bowl with red onion. Cover; set aside.

2. Rinse scallops. Cut in half horizontally (to make 2 thin rounds); pat dry. Sprinkle top side lightly with red pepper and paprika. Spray large nonstick skillet with cooking spray; heat over high heat until very hot. Add half of scallops, seasoned side down, in single layer, placing ½ inch or more apart. Sprinkle with red pepper and paprika. Cook 2 minutes or until browned on bottom. Turn scallops; cook 1 to 2 minutes or until opaque in center. Transfer to plate; cover to keep warm. Wipe skillet clean; repeat procedure with remaining scallops.

3. Place dressing in small saucepan; bring to a boil over high heat. Pour dressing over spinach and onion; toss to coat. Divide among 4 plates. Place scallops on top of spinach; sprinkle with blue cheese and walnuts.

*Makes 4 servings*

**Nutrients per Serving:** Calories: 169 (29% Calories from Fat), Total Fat: 6 g, Saturated Fat: 2 g, Protein: 24 g, Carbohydrate: 6 g, Cholesterol: 50 mg, Sodium: 660 mg, Fiber: 2 g, Sugar: trace
**Dietary Exchanges:** 3 Lean Meat, 1 Vegetable

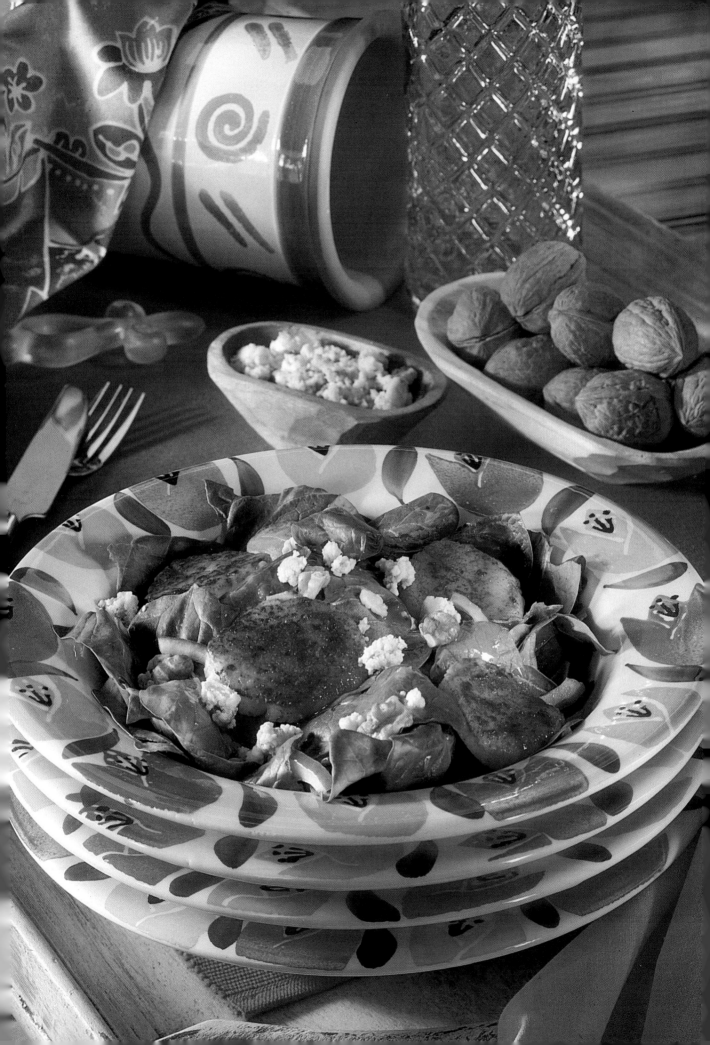

# Moroccan Lentil & Vegetable Soup

*Not only do lentils taste good, but they are also high in soluble fiber, which lowers blood cholesterol.*

**1 tablespoon olive oil**
**1 cup chopped onion**
**4 medium cloves garlic, minced**
**½ cup dry lentils, sorted, rinsed and drained**
**1½ teaspoons ground coriander**
**1½ teaspoons ground cumin**
**½ teaspoon black pepper**
**½ teaspoon ground cinnamon**
**3¾ cups fat-free reduced-sodium chicken broth**
**½ cup chopped celery**
**½ cup chopped sun-dried tomatoes (not packed in oil)**
**1 medium yellow summer squash, chopped**
**½ cup chopped green bell pepper**
**½ cup chopped parsley**
**1 cup chopped plum tomatoes**
**¼ cup chopped cilantro or basil**

1. Heat oil in medium saucepan over medium heat. Add onion and garlic; cook 4 to 5 minutes or until onion is tender, stirring occasionally. Stir in lentils, coriander, cumin, black pepper and cinnamon; cook 2 minutes. Add chicken broth, celery and sun-dried tomatoes; bring to a boil over high heat. Reduce heat to low; simmer, covered, 25 minutes.

2. Stir in squash, bell pepper and parsley. Continue cooking, covered, 10 minutes or until lentils are tender.

3. Top with plum tomatoes and cilantro just before serving.

*Makes 6 servings*

**Nutrients per Serving:** Calories: 131 (20% Calories from Fat), Total Fat: 3 g, Saturated Fat: trace, Protein: 8 g, Carbohydrate: 20 g, Cholesterol: 0 mg, Sodium: 264 mg, Fiber: 2 g, Sugar: 2 g
**Dietary Exchanges:** 1 Starch/Bread, 1 Vegetable, ½ Fat

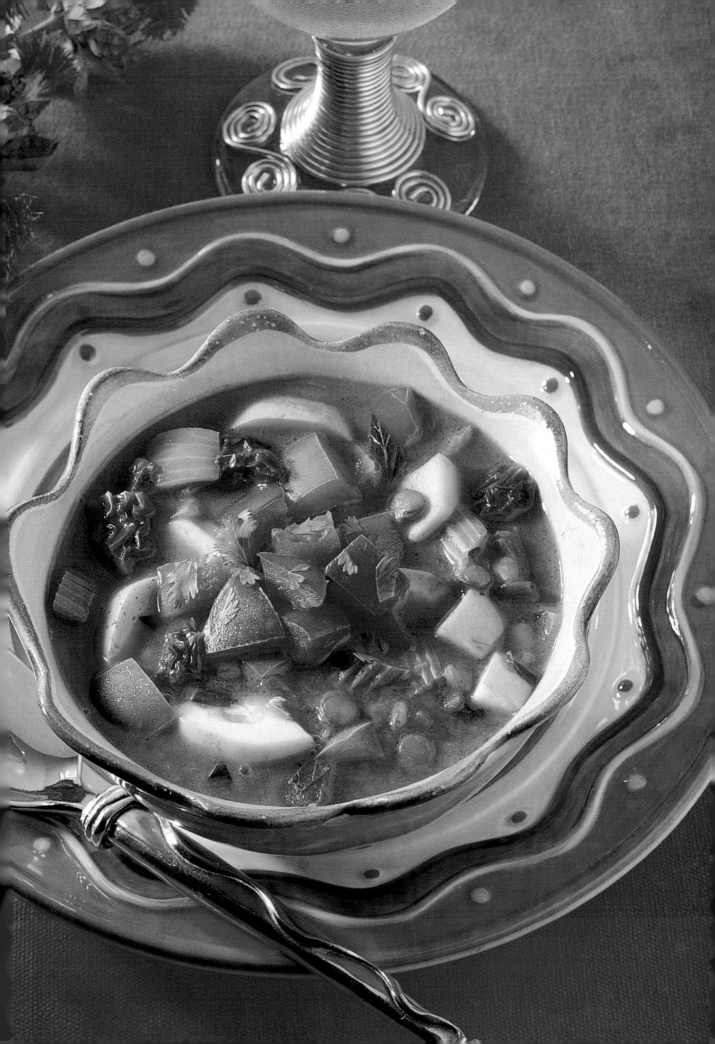

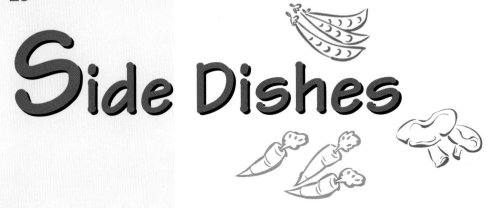

# Side Dishes

## Spicy Chick-Peas & Couscous

*Couscous is a grain-like semolina pasta used in northern African cuisines.*

    1 can (about 14 ounces) vegetable broth
    1 teaspoon ground coriander
    ½ teaspoon ground cardamom
    ½ teaspoon turmeric
    ½ teaspoon hot pepper sauce
    ¼ teaspoon salt
    ⅛ teaspoon cinnamon
    1 cup julienned carrots
    1 can (15 ounces) chick-peas, rinsed and drained
    1 cup frozen peas
    1 cup quick-cooking couscous
    2 tablespoons chopped fresh mint or parsley

1. Combine vegetable broth, coriander, cardamom, turmeric, pepper sauce, salt and cinnamon in large saucepan; bring to a boil over high heat. Add carrots; reduce heat and simmer 5 minutes. Add chick-peas and peas; return to a simmer. Simmer, uncovered, 2 minutes.

2. Stir in couscous. Cover; remove from heat. Let stand 5 minutes or until liquid is absorbed. Sprinkle with mint. *Makes 6 servings*

**Nutrients per Serving:** Calories: 226 (6% Calories from Fat), Total Fat: 2 g, Saturated Fat: trace, Protein: 9 g, Carbohydrate: 44 g, Cholesterol: 0 mg, Sodium: 431 mg, Fiber: 10 g, Sugar: 3 g
**Dietary Exchanges:** 3 Starch/Bread

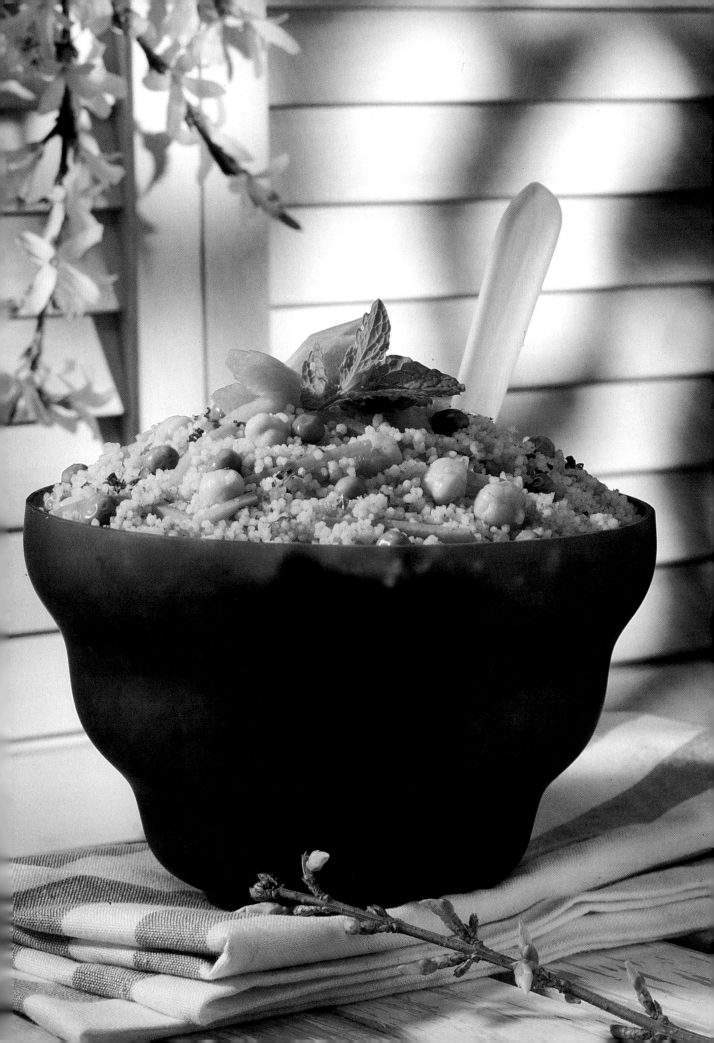

# Zucchini Shanghai Style

     4 dried Chinese black mushrooms
   1/2 cup fat-free reduced-sodium chicken broth
     2 tablespoons ketchup
     2 teaspoons dry sherry
     1 teaspoon low-sodium soy sauce
     1 teaspoon red wine vinegar
   1/4 teaspoon sugar
  1 1/2 teaspoons vegetable oil, divided
     1 teaspoon minced fresh ginger
     1 clove garlic, minced
     1 large tomato, peeled, seeded and chopped
     1 green onion, finely chopped
     4 tablespoons water, divided
     1 teaspoon cornstarch
     1 pound zucchini (about 3 medium), diagonally cut into 1-inch pieces
   1/2 small yellow onion, cut into wedges and separated

1. Soak mushrooms in warm water 20 minutes. Drain, reserving 1/4 cup liquid. Squeeze out excess water. Discard stems; slice caps. Combine reserved 1/4 cup mushroom liquid, chicken broth, ketchup, sherry, soy sauce, vinegar and sugar in small bowl. Set aside.

2. Heat 1 teaspoon oil in large saucepan over medium heat. Add ginger and garlic; stir-fry 10 seconds. Add mushrooms, tomato and green onion; stir-fry 1 minute. Add chicken broth mixture; bring to a boil over high heat. Reduce heat to medium; simmer 10 minutes.

3. Combine 1 tablespoon water and cornstarch in small bowl; set aside. Heat remaining 1/2 teaspoon oil in large nonstick skillet over medium heat. Add zucchini and yellow onion; stir-fry 30 seconds. Add remaining 3 tablespoons water. Cover and cook 3 to 4 minutes or until vegetables are crisp-tender, stirring occasionally. Add tomato mixture to skillet. Stir cornstarch mixture and add to skillet. Cook until sauce boils and thickens.

*Makes 4 servings*

**Nutrients per Serving:** Calories: 72 (23% Calories from Fat), Total Fat: 2 g, Saturated Fat: trace, Protein: 3 g, Carbohydrate: 12 g, Cholesterol: 0 mg, Sodium: 156 mg, Fiber: 3 g, Sugar: 3 g
**Dietary Exchanges:** 2 Vegetable, 1 Fat

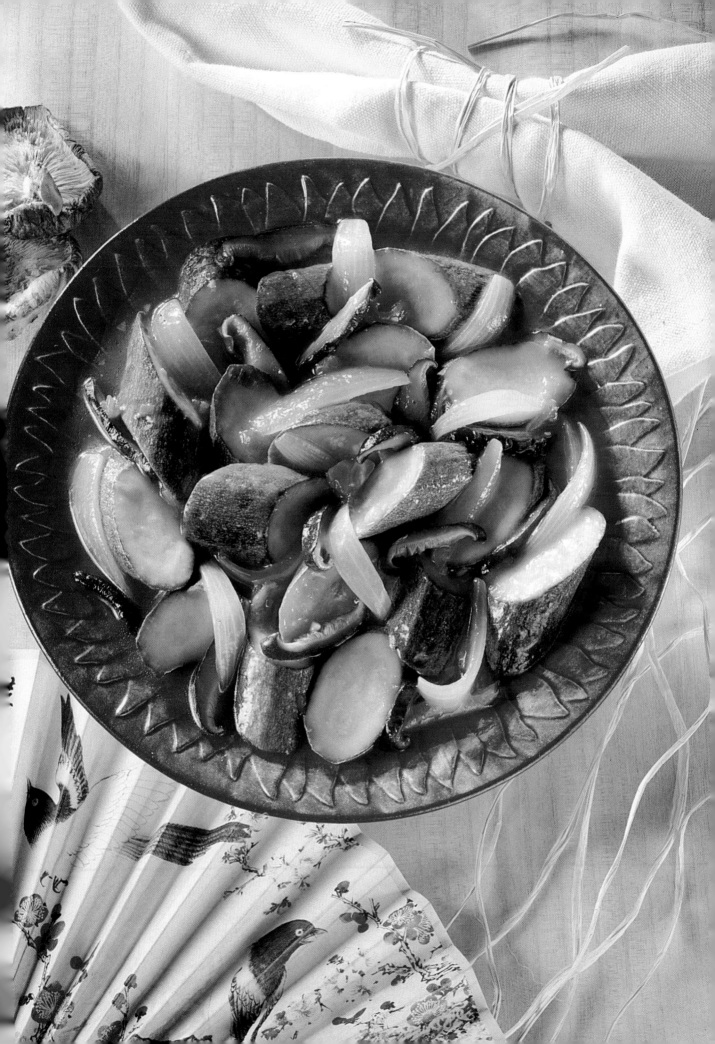

# Glazed Maple Acorn Squash

*Although acorn squash is considered a winter squash, it is usually available year round. Look for golden acorn squash, which is similar in all respects to the typical green acorn squash, but its shell has a dramatic pumpkin color.*

> **1 large acorn or golden acorn squash**
> **¼ cup water**
> **2 tablespoons pure maple syrup**
> **1 tablespoon margarine or butter, melted**
> **¼ teaspoon cinnamon**

1. Preheat oven to 375°F.

2. Cut stem and blossom ends from squash. Cut squash crosswise into four equal slices. Discard seeds and membrane. Place water in 13×9-inch baking dish. Arrange squash in dish; cover with foil. Bake 30 minutes or until tender.

3. Combine syrup, margarine and cinnamon in small bowl; mix well. Uncover squash; pour off water. Brush squash with syrup mixture, letting excess pool in center of squash.

4. Return to oven; bake 10 minutes or until syrup mixture is bubbly.

*Makes 4 servings*

**Nutrients per Serving:** Calories: 161 (16% Calories from Fat), Total Fat: 3 g, Saturated Fat: 2 g, Protein: 2 g, Carbohydrate: 35 g, Cholesterol: 8 mg, Sodium: 39 mg, Fiber: 4 g, Sugar: 14 g
**Dietary Exchanges:** 2 Starch/Bread, ½ Fat

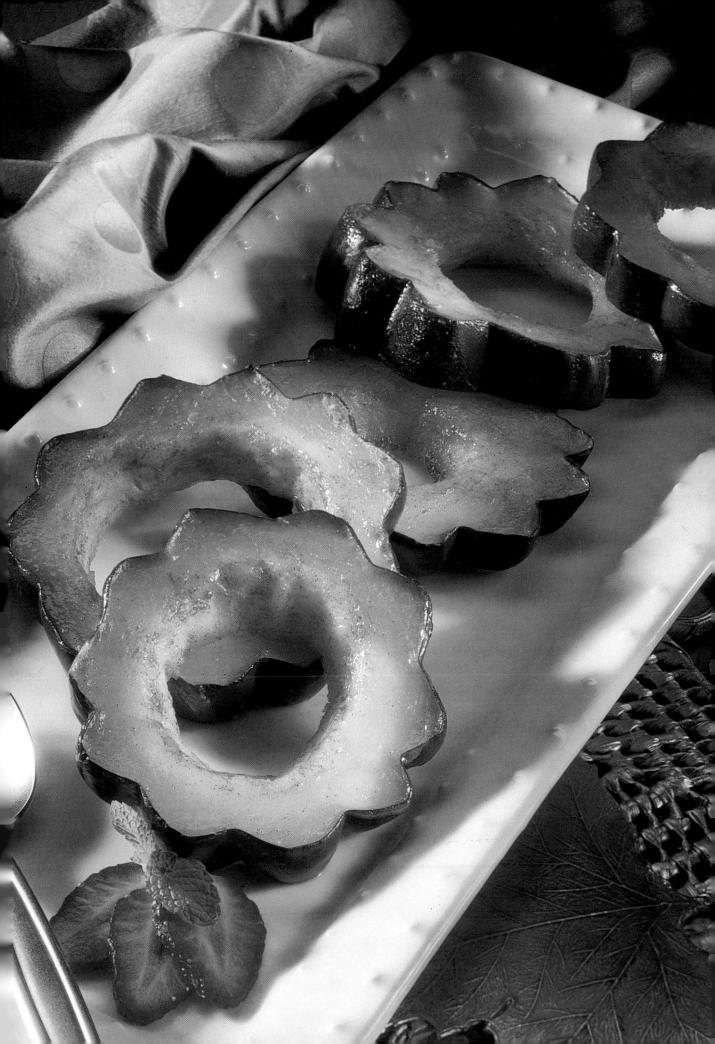

# Spicy Sesame Noodles

*Soba is a Japanese noodle made from buckwheat flour with a taste and texture that are different from the kind of spaghetti familiar to most Americans.*

6 ounces uncooked dry soba (buckwheat) noodles
2 teaspoons dark sesame oil
1 tablespoon sesame seeds
½ cup fat-free reduced-sodium chicken broth
1 tablespoon creamy peanut butter
4 teaspoons light soy sauce
½ cup thinly sliced green onions
½ cup minced red bell pepper
1½ teaspoons finely chopped, seeded jalapeño pepper*
1 clove garlic, minced
¼ teaspoon red pepper flakes

*Jalapeño peppers can sting and irritate the skin; wear rubber gloves when handling peppers and do not touch eyes. Wash hands after handling.

1. Cook noodles according to package directions. (Do not overcook.) Rinse noodles thoroughly with cold water to stop cooking and remove salty residue; drain. Place noodles in large bowl; toss with sesame oil.

2. Place sesame seeds in small skillet. Cook over medium heat about 3 minutes or until seeds begin to pop and turn golden brown, stirring frequently. Remove from heat; set aside.

3. Combine chicken broth and peanut butter in small bowl with wire whisk until blended. (Mixture may look curdled.) Stir in soy sauce, green onions, bell pepper, jalapeño pepper, garlic and red pepper flakes.

4. Pour mixture over noodles; toss to coat. Cover and let stand 30 minutes at room temperature or refrigerate up to 24 hours. Sprinkle with toasted sesame seeds before serving. *Makes 6 servings*

**Nutrients per Serving:** Calories: 145 (23% Calories from Fat), Total Fat: 4 g, Saturated Fat: 1 g, Protein: 6 g, Carbohydrate: 24 g, Cholesterol: 0 mg, Sodium: 358 mg, Fiber: 1 g, Sugar: 1 g
**Dietary Exchanges:** 1½ Starch/Bread, ½ Vegetable, ½ Fat

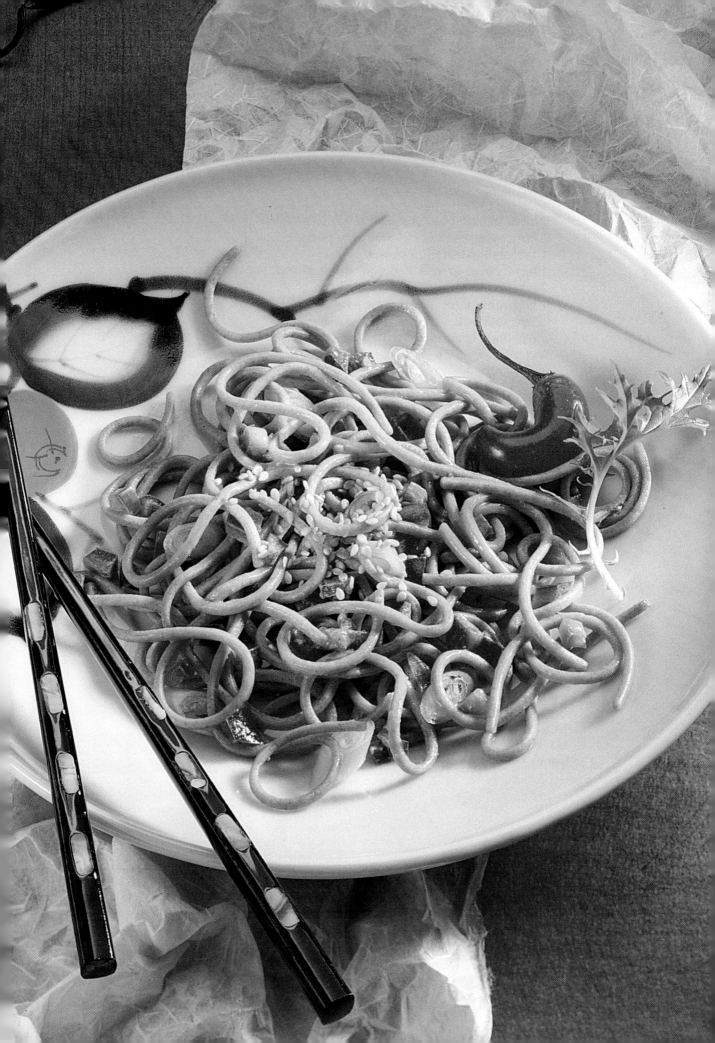

# Gratin of Two Potatoes

*This delicious side dish can be prepared up to 2 hours before baking. Let stand, covered with foil, at room temperature.*

> **2 large baking potatoes (about 1¼ pounds)**
> **2 large sweet potatoes (about 1¼ pounds)**
> **1 tablespoon unsalted butter**
> **1 large sweet or yellow onion, thinly sliced, separated into rings**
> **2 teaspoons all-purpose flour**
> **1 cup canned fat-free reduced-sodium chicken broth**
> **½ teaspoon salt**
> **¼ teaspoon ground white pepper *or* ⅛ teaspoon ground red pepper**
> **¾ cup freshly grated Parmesan cheese**

1. Cook baking potatoes in large pot of boiling water 10 minutes. Add sweet potatoes; return to a boil. Simmer potatoes, uncovered, 25 minutes or until tender. Drain; cool under cold running water.

2. Meanwhile, melt butter in large nonstick skillet over medium-high heat. Add onion; cover and cook 3 minutes or until wilted. Uncover; cook over medium-low heat 10 to 12 minutes or until tender, stirring occasionally. Sprinkle with flour; cook 1 minute, stirring frequently. Add chicken broth, salt and pepper; bring to a boil over high heat. Reduce heat to medium; simmer, uncovered, 2 minutes or until sauce thickens, stirring occasionally.

3. Preheat oven to 375°F. Spray 13×9-inch baking dish with nonstick cooking spray. Peel potatoes; cut crosswise into ¼-inch slices. Layer half of baking and sweet potato slices in prepared dish. Spoon half of onion mixture evenly over potatoes. Repeat layering with remaining potatoes and onion mixture. Cover with foil. Bake 25 minutes or until heated through.

4. Preheat broiler. Uncover potatoes; sprinkle evenly with cheese. Broil, 5 inches from heat, 3 to 4 minutes or until cheese is bubbly and light golden brown.                                                    *Makes 6 servings*

**Nutrients per Serving:** Calories: 261 (21% Calories from Fat), Total Fat: 6 g,
Saturated Fat: 4 g, Protein: 9 g, Carbohydrate: 43 g, Cholesterol: 15 mg,
Sodium: 437 mg, Fiber: 1 g, Sugar: 1 g
**Dietary Exchanges:** 3 Starch/Bread, ½ Lean Meat, ½ Fat

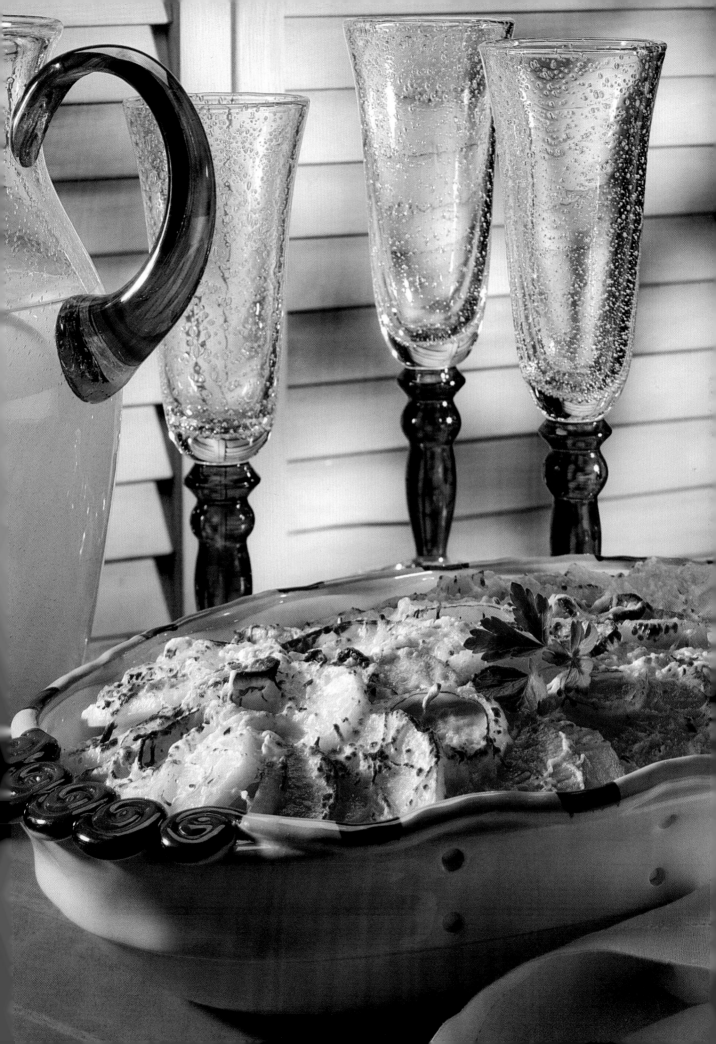

# Mediterranean-Style Roasted Vegetables

*This colorful side dish is a perfect accompaniment to grilled chicken or pork.*

1½ **pounds red potatoes**
1 **tablespoon plus 1½ teaspoons olive oil, divided**
1 **red bell pepper**
1 **yellow or orange bell pepper**
1 **small red onion**
2 **cloves garlic, minced**
½ **teaspoon salt**
¼ **teaspoon black pepper**
1 **tablespoon balsamic vinegar**
¼ **cup chopped fresh basil leaves**

1. Preheat oven to 425°F. Spray large shallow metal roasting pan with nonstick cooking spray. Cut potatoes into 1½-inch chunks; place in pan. Drizzle 1 tablespoon oil over potatoes; toss to coat. Bake 10 minutes.

2. Cut bell peppers into 1½-inch chunks. Cut onion through the core into ½-inch wedges. Add bell peppers and onion to pan. Drizzle remaining 1½ teaspoons oil over vegetables; sprinkle with garlic, salt and black pepper. Toss well to coat. Return to oven; bake 18 to 20 minutes or until vegetables are brown and tender, stirring once.

3. Transfer to large serving bowl. Drizzle vinegar over vegetables; toss to coat. Add basil; toss again. Serve warm or at room temperature with additional black pepper, if desired.           *Makes 6 servings*

**Nutrients per Serving:** Calories: 170 (19% Calories from Fat), Total Fat: 4 g, Saturated Fat: trace, Protein: 3 g, Carbohydrate: 33 g, Cholesterol: 0 mg, Sodium: 185 mg, Fiber: 1 g, Sugar: trace
**Dietary Exchanges:** 2 Starch/Bread, ½ Fat

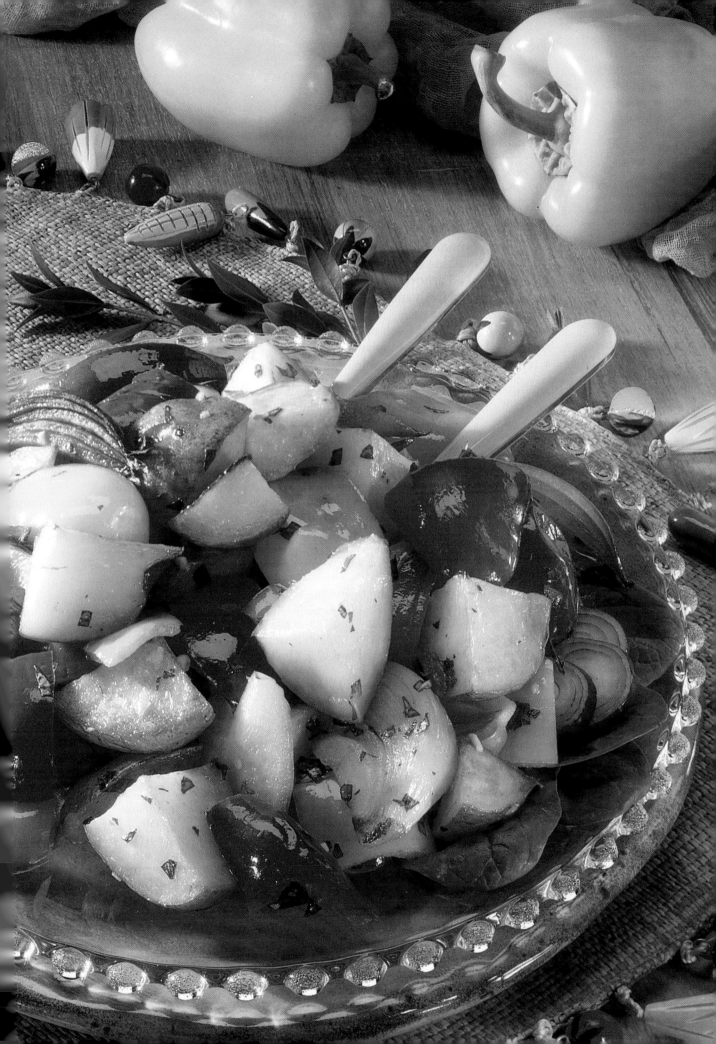

# Spinach Parmesan Risotto

*Arborio rice, an Italian-grown short-grain rice, has large, plump grains with a delicious nutty taste. It is traditionally used for risotto dishes because its high starch content produces a creamy texture.*

  3²/₃ **cups fat-free reduced-sodium chicken broth**
   ½ **teaspoon ground white pepper**
      **Nonstick cooking spray**
    1 **cup uncooked arborio rice**
  1½ **cups chopped fresh spinach**
   ½ **cup frozen green peas**
    1 **tablespoon minced fresh dill** *or* **1 teaspoon dried dill weed**
   ½ **cup grated Parmesan cheese**
    1 **teaspoon grated lemon peel**

1. Combine chicken broth and pepper in medium saucepan; cover. Bring to a simmer over medium-low heat; maintain simmer by adjusting heat.

2. Spray large saucepan with cooking spray; heat over medium-low heat. Add rice; cook and stir 1 minute. Stir in ²/₃ cup hot chicken broth; cook, stirring constantly until chicken broth is absorbed.

3. Stir remaining hot chicken broth into rice mixture, ½ cup at a time, stirring constantly until all chicken broth is absorbed before adding next ½ cup. When adding last ½ cup chicken broth, stir in spinach, peas and dill. Cook, stirring gently until all chicken broth is absorbed and rice is just tender but still firm to the bite. (Total cooking time for chicken broth absorption is 35 to 40 minutes.)

4. Remove saucepan from heat; stir in cheese and lemon peel.

*Makes 6 servings*

**Nutrients per Serving:** Calories: 179 (15% Calories from Fat), Total Fat: 3 g, Saturated Fat: 2 g, Protein: 7 g, Carbohydrate: 30 g, Cholesterol: 7 mg, Sodium: 198 mg, Fiber: 1 g, Sugar: 1 g
**Dietary Exchanges:** 2 Starch/Bread, ½ Lean Meat

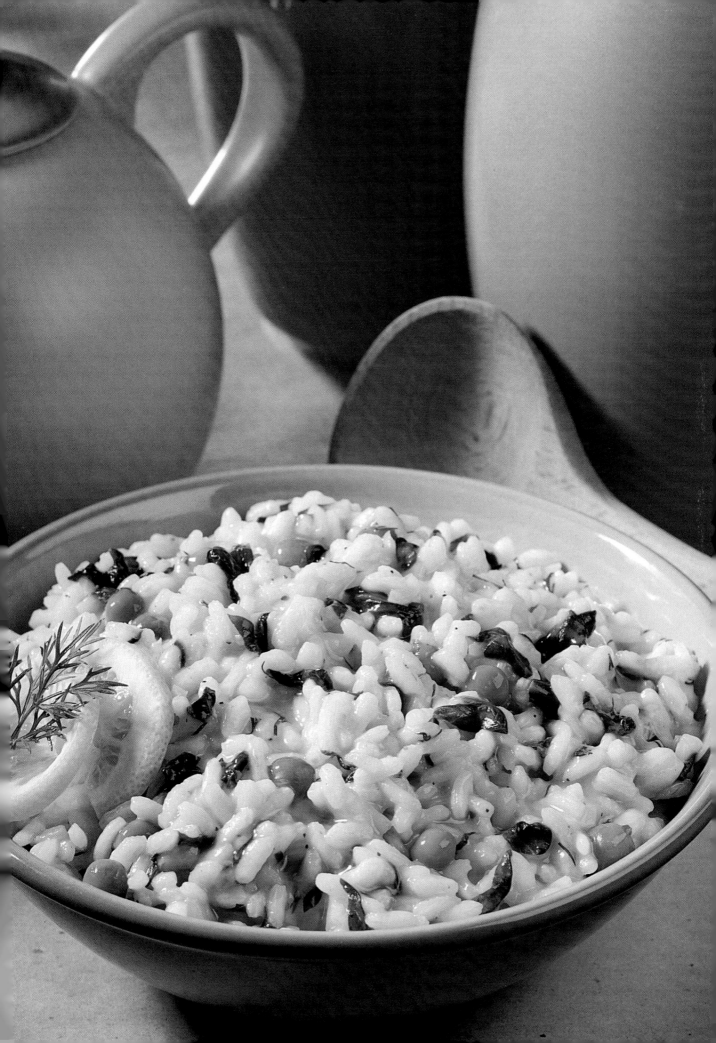

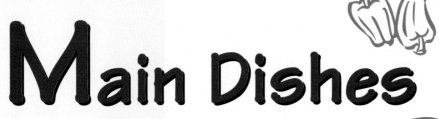

# Main Dishes

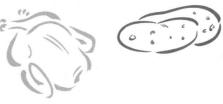

## Roast Chicken & Potatoes Catalan

**2 tablespoons olive oil**
**2 tablespoons lemon juice**
**1 teaspoon dried thyme leaves**
**½ teaspoon salt**
**¼ teaspoon ground red pepper**
**¼ teaspoon ground saffron** *or* **½ teaspoon crushed saffron threads or turmeric**
**2 large baking potatoes (about 1½ pounds), cut into 1½-inch chunks**
**4 skinless bone-in chicken breast halves (about 2 pounds)**
**1 cup sliced red bell pepper**
**1 cup frozen peas, thawed**
**Lemon wedges**

1. Preheat oven to 400°F. Spray large shallow roasting pan or 15×10-inch jelly-roll pan with nonstick cooking spray.

2. Combine oil, lemon juice, thyme, salt, ground red pepper and saffron in large bowl; mix well. Add potatoes; toss to coat.

3. Arrange potatoes in single layer around edges of pan. Place chicken in center of pan; brush both sides of chicken with remaining oil mixture in bowl.

4. Bake 20 minutes. Turn potatoes; baste chicken with pan juices. Add bell pepper; continue baking 20 minutes or until chicken is no longer pink in center, juices run clear and potatoes are browned. Stir peas into potato mixture; bake 5 minutes or until heated through. Garnish with lemon wedges. *Makes 4 servings*

**Nutrients per Serving:** Calories: 541 (18% Calories from Fat), Total Fat: 11 g, Saturated Fat: 2 g, Protein: 42 g, Carbohydrate: 69 g, Cholesterol: 91 mg, Sodium: 132 mg, Fiber: 3 g, Sugar: 2 g
**Dietary Exchanges:** 4 Starch/Bread, 4 Lean Meat, 1 Vegetable

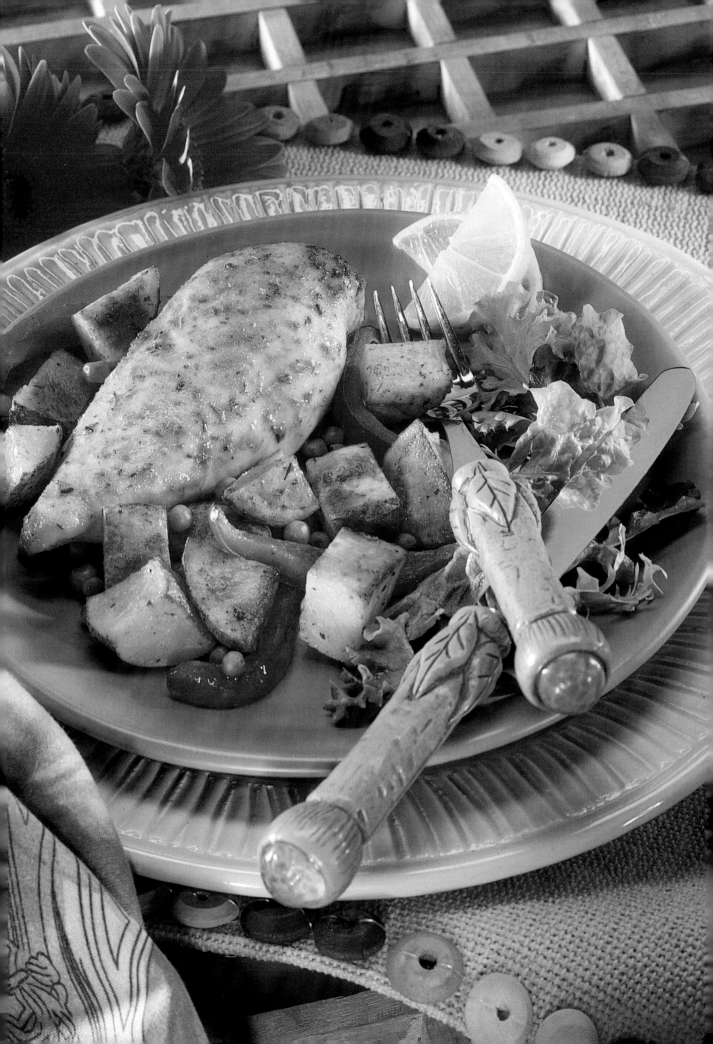

# Mushroom Ragoût with Polenta

*This easy meatless main dish will please the whole family. Cooking the polenta in the microwave oven is foolproof and makes cleanup easy.*

**1 package (about ½ ounce) dried porcini mushrooms**
**½ cup boiling water**
**1 can (about 14 ounces) vegetable broth**
**½ cup yellow cornmeal**
**1 tablespoon olive oil**
**⅓ cup sliced shallots or chopped sweet onion**
**1 package (4 ounces) sliced mixed fresh exotic mushrooms or sliced cremini mushrooms**
**4 cloves garlic, minced**
**1 can (14½ ounces) Italian-style diced tomatoes, undrained**
**¼ teaspoon red pepper flakes**
**¼ cup chopped fresh basil or parsley**
**½ cup grated fat-free Parmesan cheese**

1. Soak porcini mushrooms in boiling water 10 minutes.

2. Meanwhile, whisk together vegetable broth and cornmeal in large microwavable bowl. Cover with waxed paper; microwave at HIGH 5 minutes. Whisk well; cook at HIGH 3 to 4 minutes or until polenta is very thick. Whisk again; cover. Set aside.

3. Heat oil in large nonstick skillet over medium-high heat. Add shallots; cook and stir 3 minutes. Add fresh mushrooms and garlic; cook and stir 3 to 4 minutes. Add tomatoes and red pepper flakes.

4. Drain porcini mushrooms; add liquid to skillet. If mushrooms are large, cut into ½-inch pieces; add to skillet. Bring to a boil over high heat. Reduce heat to medium; simmer, uncovered, 5 minutes or until slightly thickened. Stir in basil.

5. Spoon polenta onto 4 plates; top with mushroom mixture. Sprinkle with cheese.                    *Makes 4 servings*

**Nutrients per Serving:** Calories: 184 (25% Calories from Fat), Total Fat: 5 g, Saturated Fat: 1 g, Protein: 6 g, Carbohydrate: 30 g, Cholesterol: 0 mg, Sodium: 572 mg, Fiber: 3 g, Sugar: 6 g
**Dietary Exchanges:** 1 Starch/Bread, ½ Lean Meat, 2½ Vegetable, ½ Fat

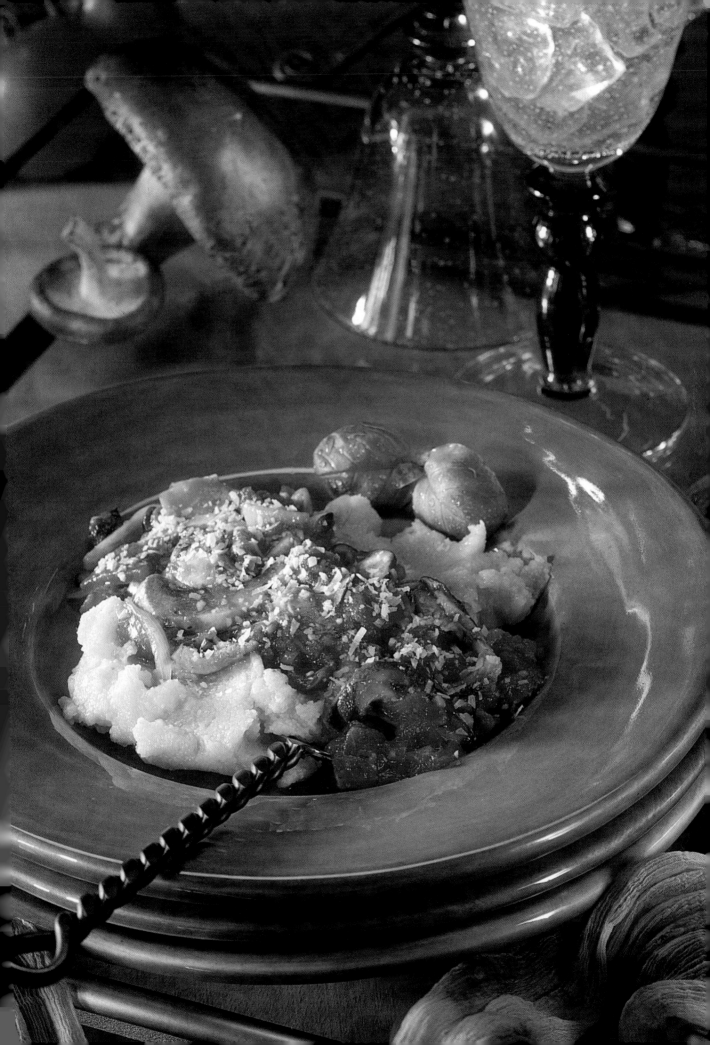

# Thai-Style Pork Kabobs

*Wooden skewers may be substituted for metal skewers. Soak them in cold water for 20 minutes to prevent them from burning during grilling.*

   $^1/_3$ **cup reduced-sodium soy sauce**
   **2 tablespoons fresh lime juice**
   **2 tablespoons water**
   **2 teaspoons hot chili oil***
   **2 cloves garlic, minced**
   **1 teaspoon minced fresh ginger**
   **12 ounces well-trimmed pork tenderloin**
   **1 red or yellow bell pepper, cut into $^1/_2$-inch chunks**
   **1 red or sweet onion, cut into $^1/_2$-inch chunks**
   **2 cups hot cooked rice**

*If hot chili oil is not available, combine 2 teaspoons vegetable oil and $^1/_2$ teaspoon red pepper flakes in small microwavable cup. Microwave at HIGH 1 minute. Let stand 5 minutes to infuse flavor.

1. Combine soy sauce, lime juice, water, chili oil, garlic and ginger in medium bowl; reserve $^1/_3$ cup mixture for dipping sauce. Set aside.

2. Cut pork tenderloin lengthwise in half; cut crosswise into 4-inch slices. Cut slices into $^1/_2$-inch strips. Add to bowl with soy sauce mixture; toss to coat. Cover; refrigerate at least 30 minutes or up to 2 hours, turning once.

3. To prevent sticking, spray grid with nonstick cooking spray. Prepare coals for grilling.

4. Remove pork from marinade; discard marinade. Alternately weave pork strips and thread bell pepper and onion chunks onto eight 8- to 10-inch metal skewers.

5. Grill, covered, over medium-hot coals 6 to 8 minutes or until pork is no longer pink in center, turning halfway through grilling time. Serve with rice and reserved dipping sauce.                      *Makes 4 servings*

**Nutrients per Serving:** Calories: 248 (16% Calories from Fat), Total Fat: 4 g, Saturated Fat: 1 g, Protein: 22 g, Carbohydrate: 30 g, Cholesterol: 49 mg, Sodium: 271 mg, Fiber: 2 g, Sugar: 1 g
**Dietary Exchanges:** 1$^1/_2$ Starch/Bread, 2 Lean Meat, 1 Vegetable

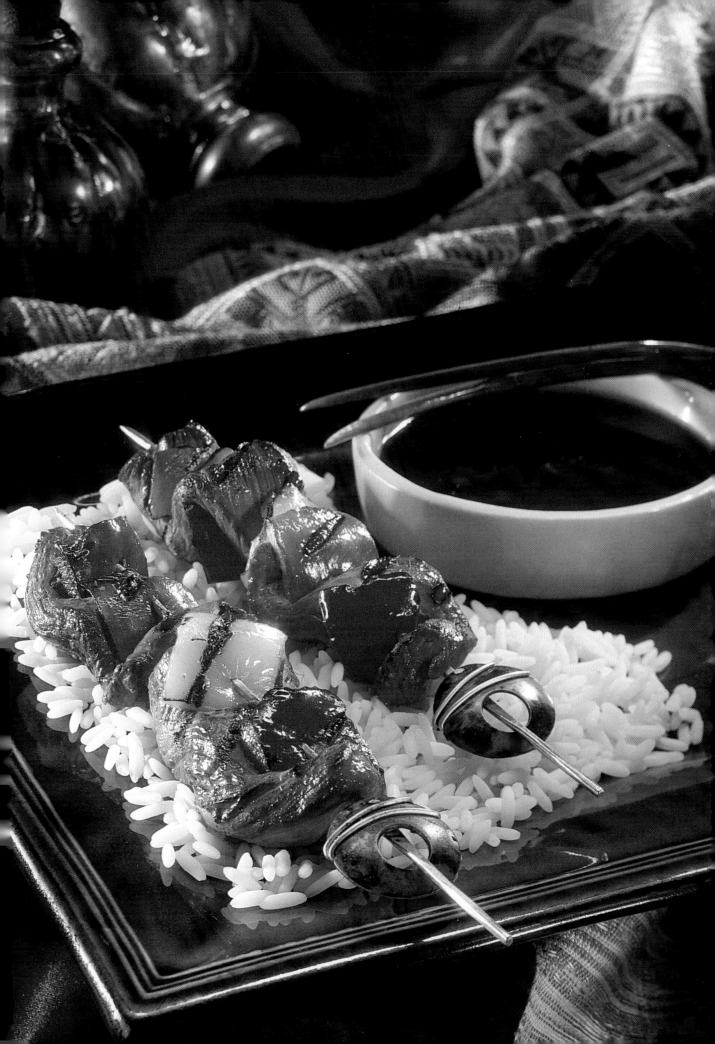

# Szechwan Beef Lo Mein

*Serve this spicy Asian one-dish meal with a chilled cucumber salad and fresh pineapple spears. Partially freezing the steak makes it easier to cut into strips.*

**1 pound well-trimmed boneless beef top sirloin steak, 1 inch thick**
**4 cloves garlic, minced**
**2 teaspoons minced fresh ginger**
**3/4 teaspoon red pepper flakes, divided**
**1 tablespoon vegetable oil**
**1 can (about 14 ounces) vegetable broth**
**1 cup water**
**2 tablespoons reduced-sodium soy sauce**
**1 package (8 ounces) frozen mixed vegetables for stir-fry**
**1 package (9 ounces) refrigerated angel hair pasta**
**1/4 cup chopped cilantro (optional)**

1. Cut steak crosswise into 1/8-inch strips; cut strips into 1 1/2-inch pieces. Toss steak with garlic, ginger and 1/2 teaspoon red pepper flakes.

2. Heat oil in large nonstick skillet over medium-high heat. Add half of steak to skillet; cook and stir 3 minutes or until meat is barely pink in center. Remove from skillet; set aside. Repeat with remaining steak.

3. Add vegetable broth, water, soy sauce and remaining 1/4 teaspoon red pepper flakes to skillet; bring to a boil over high heat. Add vegetables; return to a boil. Reduce heat to low; simmer, covered, 3 minutes or until vegetables are crisp-tender.

4. Uncover; stir in pasta. Return to a boil over high heat. Reduce heat to medium; simmer, uncovered, 2 minutes, separating pasta with two forks. Return steak and any accumulated juices to skillet; simmer 1 minute or until pasta is tender and steak is hot. Sprinkle with cilantro, if desired.

*Makes 4 servings*

**Nutrients per Serving:** Calories: 408 (25% Calories from Fat), Total Fat: 11 g, Saturated Fat: 3 g, Protein: 32 g, Carbohydrate: 44 g, Cholesterol: 137 mg, Sodium: 386 mg, Fiber: 2 g, Sugar: 1 g
**Dietary Exchanges:** 2 Starch/Bread, 3 Lean Meat, 3 Vegetable, 1/2 Fat

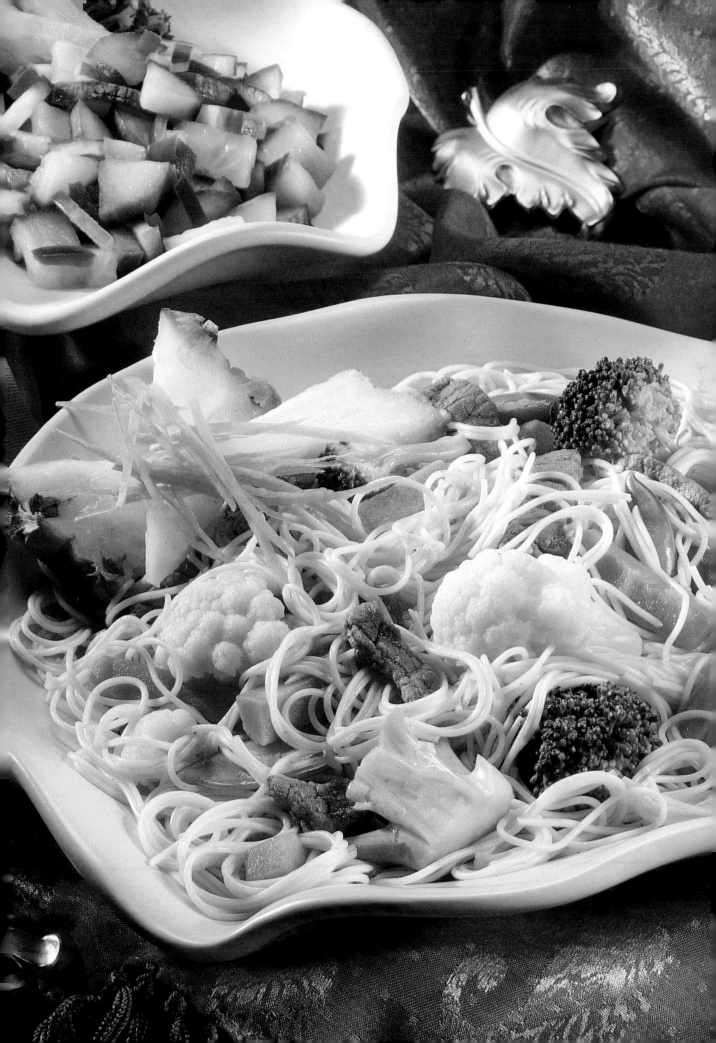

# Broiled Caribbean Sea Bass

*This flavorful fish entrée needs only 30 minutes to marinate and cooks quickly. The black bean and rice mix provides a quick yet authentic accompaniment to the fish.*

**6 skinless sea bass or striped bass fillets (5 to 6 ounces each), about ½ inch thick**
**⅓ cup chopped cilantro**
**2 tablespoons olive oil**
**2 tablespoons fresh lime juice**
**2 teaspoons hot pepper sauce**
**2 cloves garlic, minced**
**1 package (7 ounces) black bean and rice mix**
**Lime wedges**

1. Place fish in shallow dish. Combine cilantro, oil, lime juice, pepper sauce and garlic in small bowl; pour over fish. Cover; marinate in refrigerator 30 minutes or up to 2 hours.

2. Prepare black bean and rice mix according to package directions; keep warm.

3. Preheat broiler. Remove fish from marinade. Place fish on rack of broiler pan; drizzle with any remaining marinade in dish. Broil, 4 to 5 inches from heat, 8 to 10 minutes or until fish is opaque. Serve with black beans and rice and lime wedges. *Makes 6 servings*

**Nutrients per Serving:** Calories: 307 (23% Calories from Fat), Total Fat: 8 g, Saturated Fat: 1 g, Protein: 33 g, Carbohydrate: 30 g, Cholesterol: 59 mg, Sodium: 432 mg, Fiber: 5 g, Sugar: 5 g
**Dietary Exchanges:** 2 Starch/Bread, 3 Lean Meat

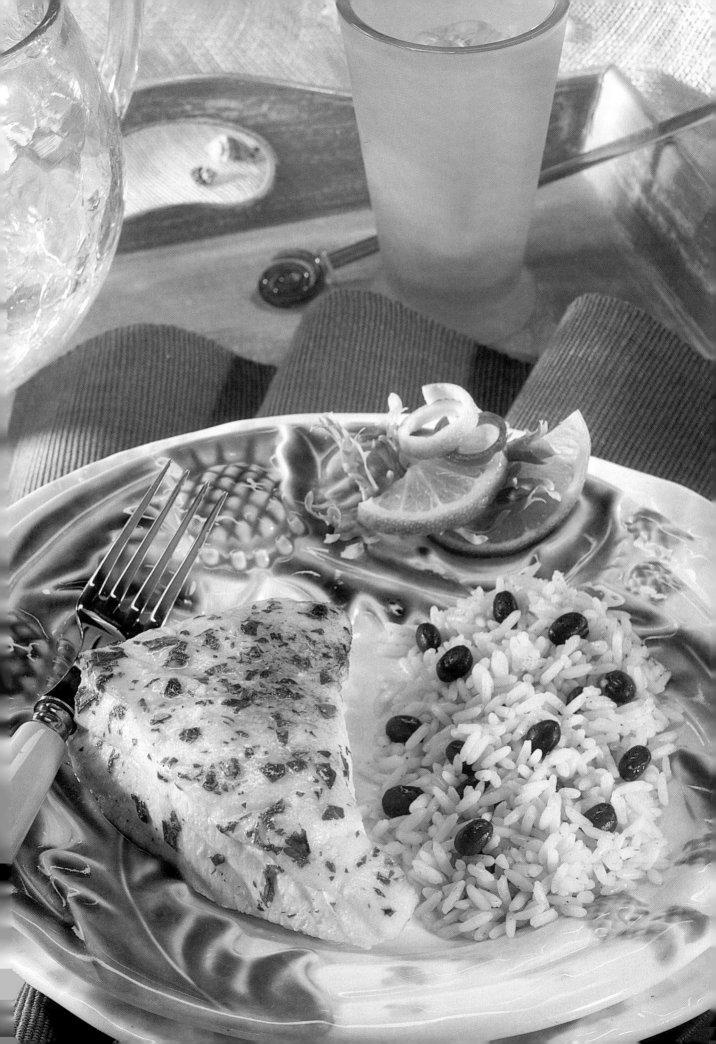

# Curried Chicken & Vegetables with Rice

*Serve this spicy curry with traditional condiments of toasted coconut and mango chutney.*

**1 pound chicken tenders or boneless skinless chicken breasts, cut crosswise into ½-inch slices**
**2 teaspoons curry powder**
**¼ teaspoon ground red pepper**
**¼ teaspoon salt**
**1 tablespoon vegetable oil**
**1 medium onion, chopped**
**3 cloves garlic, minced**
**1¼ cups canned fat-free reduced-sodium chicken broth, divided**
**2 tablespoons tomato paste**
**1 package (16 ounces) frozen mixed vegetable medley, such as broccoli, red bell peppers, cauliflower and sugar snap peas, thawed**
**2 teaspoons cornstarch**
**3 cups hot cooked white rice**
**½ cup plain nonfat yogurt**
**⅓ cup chopped cilantro**

1. Toss chicken with curry powder, ground red pepper and salt in medium bowl; set aside.

2. Heat oil in large skillet over medium heat. Add onion; cook 5 minutes, stirring occasionally. Add chicken and garlic; cook 4 minutes or until chicken is no longer pink in center, stirring occasionally. Add 1 cup chicken broth, tomato paste and vegetables; bring to a boil over high heat. Reduce heat to medium; simmer, uncovered, 3 to 4 minutes or until vegetables are crisp-tender.

3. Combine remaining ¼ cup chicken broth and cornstarch, mixing until smooth. Stir into chicken mixture; simmer 2 minutes or until sauce thickens, stirring occasionally. Serve over rice; top with yogurt and cilantro. *Makes 4 servings*

**Nutrients per Serving:** Calories: 404 (16% Calories from Fat), Total Fat: 7 g, Saturated Fat: 1 g, Protein: 34 g, Carbohydrate: 50 g, Cholesterol: 69 mg, Sodium: 299 mg, Fiber: 4 g, Sugar: 2 g
**Dietary Exchanges:** 2½ Starch/Bread, 3 Lean Meat, 2 Vegetable

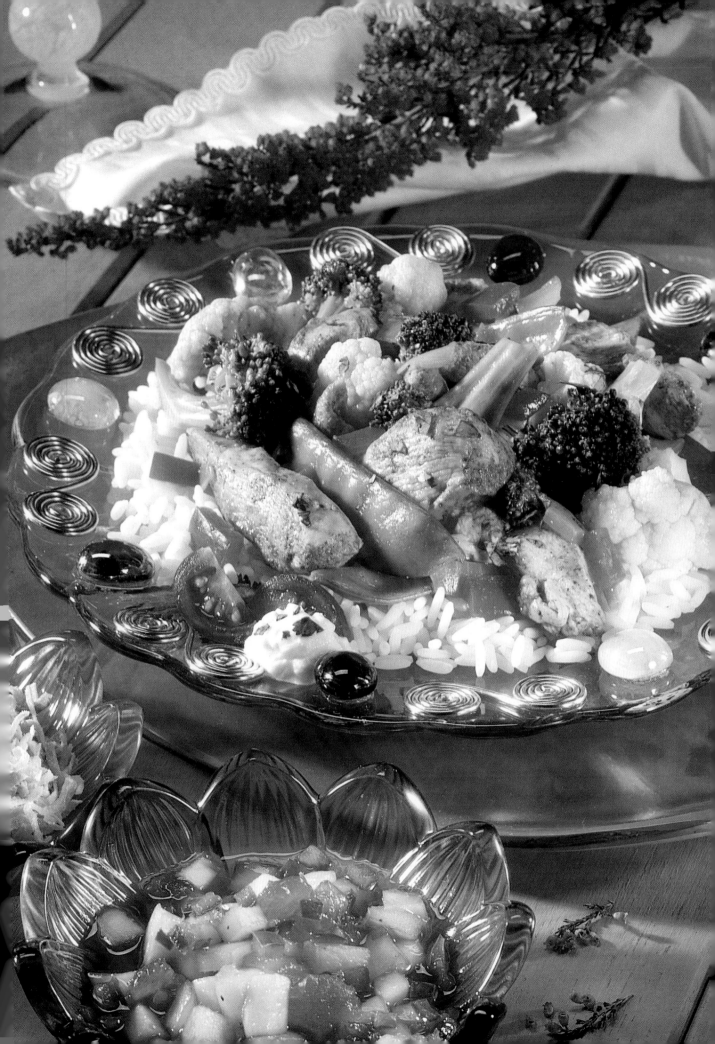

# Chipotle Tamale Pie

*Chipotle chilies are smoked jalapeño peppers. Look for cans of smoky hot chipotle chilies in the ethnic section of your supermarket.*

¾ **pound ground turkey breast or lean ground beef**
1 **cup chopped onion**
¾ **cup diced green bell pepper**
¾ **cup diced red bell pepper**
4 **cloves garlic, minced**
2 **teaspoons ground cumin**
1 **can (15 ounces) pinto or red beans, rinsed and drained**
1 **can (8 ounces) no-salt-added stewed tomatoes, undrained**
2 **canned chipotle chilies in adobo sauce, minced (about**
    1 **tablespoon)**
1 **to 2 teaspoons adobo sauce from canned chilies (optional)**
1 **cup (4 ounces) low-sodium reduced-fat shredded Cheddar cheese**
½ **cup chopped cilantro**
1 **package (8½ ounces) corn bread mix**
⅓ **cup 1% low-fat milk**
1 **large egg white**

1. Preheat oven to 400°F.

2. Cook turkey, onion, bell peppers and garlic in large nonstick skillet over medium-high heat 8 minutes or until turkey is no longer pink, stirring occasionally. Drain fat; sprinkle mixture with cumin.

3. Add beans, tomatoes, chilies and adobo sauce; bring to a boil over high heat. Reduce heat to medium; simmer, uncovered, 5 minutes. Remove from heat; stir in cheese and cilantro.

4. Spray 8-inch square baking dish with nonstick cooking spray. Spoon turkey mixture evenly into prepared dish, pressing down to compact mixture. Combine corn bread mix, milk and egg white in medium bowl; mix just until dry ingredients are moistened. Spoon batter evenly over turkey mixture to cover completely.

5. Bake 20 to 22 minutes or until corn bread is golden brown. Let stand 5 minutes before serving.                                *Makes 6 servings*

**Nutrients per Serving:** Calories: 396 (23% Calories from Fat), Total Fat: 10 g, Saturated Fat: 3 g, Protein: 26 g, Carbohydrate: 52 g, Cholesterol: 32 mg, Sodium: 733 mg, Fiber: 2 g, Sugar: 3 g
**Dietary Exchanges:** 3 Starch/Bread, 2 Lean Meat, 1½ Vegetable, ½ Fat

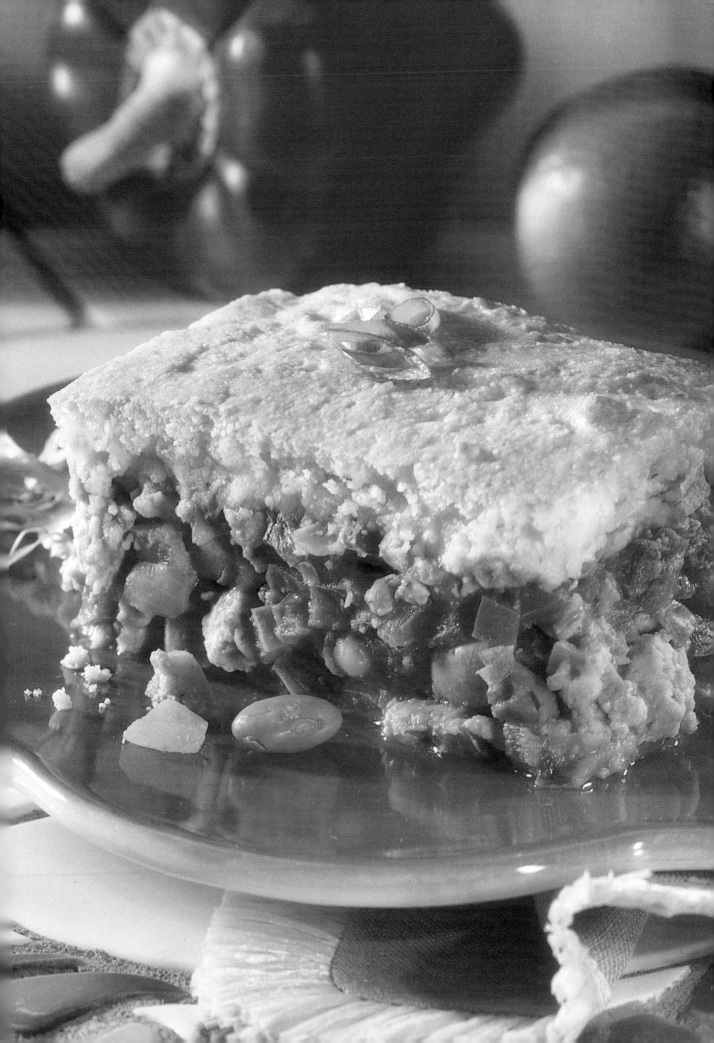

# Latin-Style Pasta & Beans

*Round out this hearty meatless main dish with warm corn tortillas and slices of melon.*

**8 ounces uncooked mostaccioli, penne or bow tie pasta**
**1 tablespoon olive oil**
**1 medium onion, chopped**
**1 yellow or red bell pepper, diced**
**4 cloves garlic, minced**
**1 can (15 ounces) red or black beans, rinsed and drained**
**¾ cup canned vegetable broth**
**¾ cup medium-hot salsa or picante sauce**
**2 teaspoons ground cumin**
**⅓ cup coarsely chopped cilantro**
**Lime wedges**

1. Cook pasta according to package directions, omitting salt. Drain; set aside.

2. Meanwhile, heat oil in a large skillet over medium heat. Add onion; cook 5 minutes, stirring occasionally. Add bell pepper and garlic; cook 3 minutes, stirring occasionally. Add beans, vegetable broth, salsa and cumin; simmer, uncovered, 5 minutes.

3. Add pasta to skillet; cook 1 minute, tossing frequently. Stir in cilantro; spoon onto 4 plates. Serve with lime wedges.            *Makes 4 servings*

**Nutrients per Serving:** Calories: 390 (12% Calories from Fat), Total Fat: 6 g, Saturated Fat: 1 g, Protein: 18 g, Carbohydrate: 74 g, Cholesterol: 0 mg, Sodium: 557 mg, Fiber: 8 g, Sugar: 1 g
**Dietary Exchanges:** 4 Starch/Bread, 1 Lean Meat, 1 Vegetable, ½ Fat

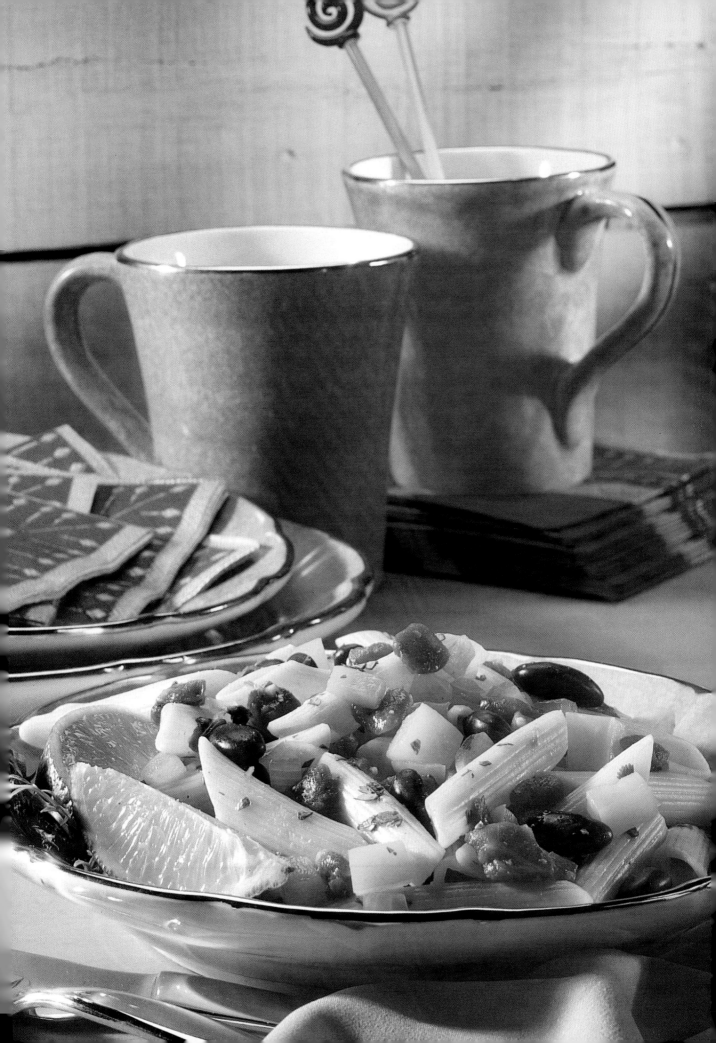

# Moroccan Pork Tagine

*Tagine is a traditional Moroccan stew typically made with chicken or lamb, vegetables and spices that is served over couscous. This tagine features pork tenderloin, which is naturally very lean and flavorful.*

> **1 pound well-trimmed pork tenderloin, cut into ¾-inch medallions**
> **1 tablespoon all-purpose flour**
> **1 teaspoon ground cumin**
> **1 teaspoon paprika**
> **¼ teaspoon powdered saffron *or* ½ teaspoon turmeric**
> **¼ teaspoon ground red pepper**
> **¼ teaspoon ground ginger**
> **1 tablespoon olive oil**
> **1 medium onion, chopped**
> **3 cloves garlic, minced**
> **2½ cups canned chicken broth, divided**
> **⅓ cup golden or dark raisins**
> **1 cup quick-cooking couscous**
> **¼ cup chopped cilantro**
> **¼ cup sliced toasted almonds (optional)**

1. Toss pork with flour, cumin, paprika, saffron, pepper and ginger in medium bowl; set aside.

2. Heat oil in large nonstick skillet over medium-high heat. Add onion; cook 5 minutes, stirring occasionally. Add pork and garlic; cook 4 to 5 minutes or until pork is no longer pink, stirring occasionally. Add ¾ cup chicken broth and raisins; bring to a boil over high heat. Reduce heat to medium; simmer, uncovered, 7 to 8 minutes or until pork is cooked through, stirring occasionally.

3. Meanwhile, bring remaining 1¾ cups chicken broth to a boil in medium saucepan. Stir in couscous. Cover; remove from heat. Let stand 5 minutes or until liquid is absorbed.

4. Spoon couscous onto 4 plates; top with pork mixture. Sprinkle with cilantro and almonds, if desired.                    *Makes 4 servings*

**Nutrients per Serving:** Calories: 435 (20% Calories from Fat), Total Fat: 10 g, Saturated Fat: 2 g, Protein: 33 g, Carbohydrate: 53 g, Cholesterol: 70 mg, Sodium: 686 mg, Fiber: 8 g, Sugar: 10 g
**Dietary Exchanges:** 2½ Starch/Bread, 3½ Lean Meat, 1 Fruit

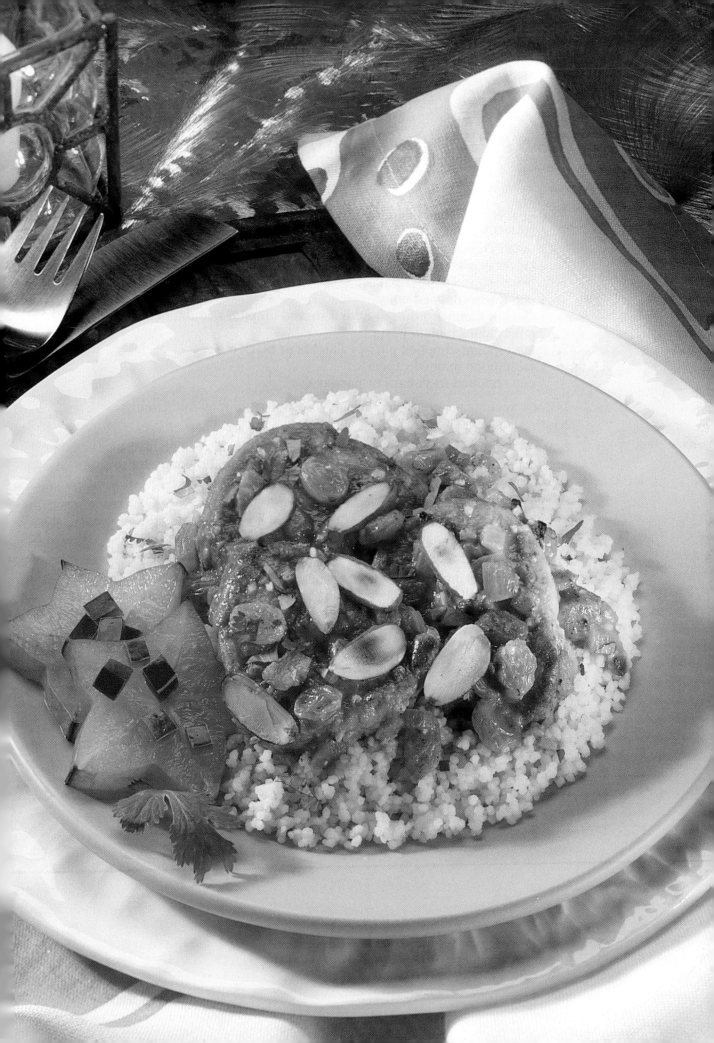

# Spicy Shrimp Puttanesca

*To save time, look for frozen peeled uncooked shrimp in the frozen food section of your supermarket.*

>     8 ounces uncooked linguine, capellini or spaghetti
>     1 tablespoon olive oil
>    12 ounces medium shrimp, peeled and deveined
>     4 cloves garlic, minced
>    ¾ teaspoon red pepper flakes
>     1 cup finely chopped onion
>     1 can (14½ ounces) no-salt-added stewed tomatoes, undrained
>     2 tablespoons tomato paste
>     2 tablespoons chopped pitted calamata or black olives
>     1 tablespoon drained capers
>    ¼ cup chopped fresh basil or parsley

1. Cook linguine according to package directions, omitting salt. Drain; set aside.

2. Meanwhile, heat oil in large nonstick skillet over medium high heat. Add shrimp, garlic and red pepper flakes; cook and stir 3 to 4 minutes or until shrimp are opaque. Transfer shrimp mixture to bowl with slotted spoon; set aside.

3. Add onion to same skillet; cook over medium heat 5 minutes, stirring occasionally. Add tomatoes, tomato paste, olives and capers; simmer, uncovered, 5 minutes.

4. Return shrimp mixture to skillet; simmer 1 minute. Stir in basil; simmer 1 minute. Place linguine in large serving bowl; top with shrimp mixture.

*Makes 4 servings*

**Nutrients per Serving:** Calories: 328 (22% Calories from Fat), Total Fat: 8 g, Saturated Fat: 1 g, Protein: 24 g, Carbohydrate: 42 g, Cholesterol: 131 mg, Sodium: 537 mg, Fiber: 2 g, Sugar: 4 g
**Dietary Exchanges:** 2 Starch/Bread, 1½ Lean Meat, 2 Vegetable, 1 Fat

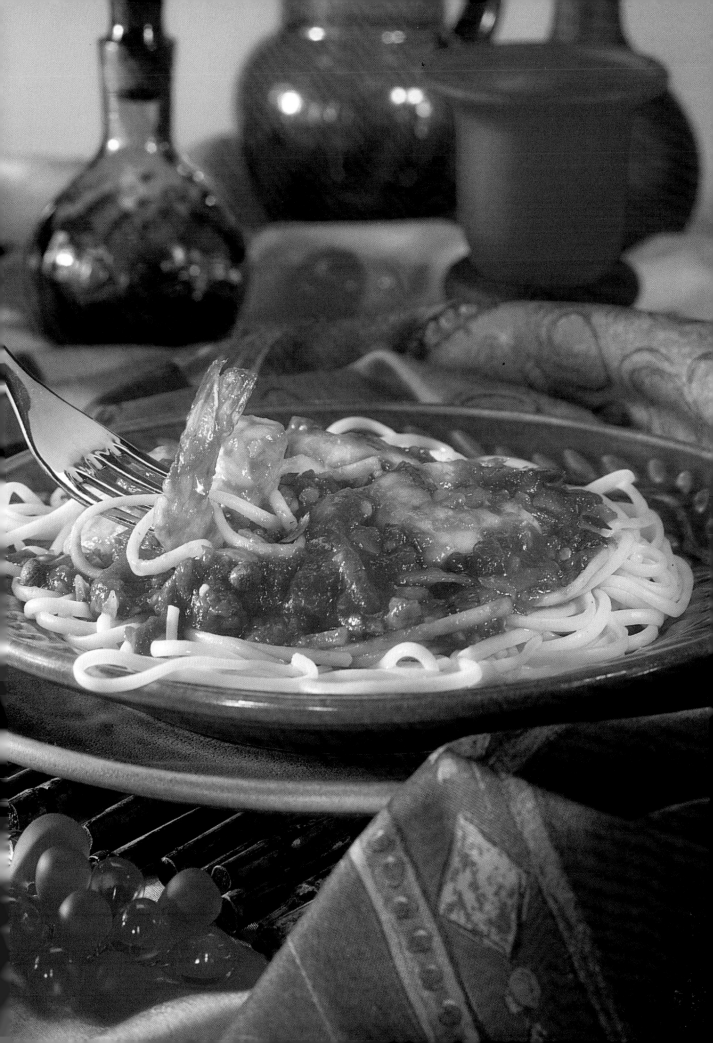

# Cajun-Style Chicken Gumbo

**1 pound boneless skinless chicken breasts**
**1 teaspoon Cajun or Creole seasoning**
**1 teaspoon dried thyme leaves**
**2 tablespoons vegetable oil**
**1 medium onion, coarsely chopped**
**1 green bell pepper, coarsely chopped**
**1 cup thinly sliced or julienned carrots**
**½ cup thinly sliced celery**
**4 cloves garlic, minced**
**2 tablespoons all-purpose flour**
**1 can (about 14 ounces) fat-free reduced-sodium chicken broth**
**1 can (14½ ounces) no-salt-added stewed tomatoes, undrained**
**½ teaspoon hot pepper sauce**
**2 cups hot cooked rice**
**¼ cup chopped parsley (optional)**
**Additional hot pepper sauce (optional)**

1. Cut chicken into 1-inch pieces; place in medium bowl. Sprinkle with seasoning and thyme; toss well. Set aside.

2. Heat oil in large saucepan over medium-high heat. Add onion, bell pepper, carrots, celery and garlic to saucepan; cover and cook 10 minutes or until vegetables are crisp-tender, stirring once. Add chicken; cook 3 minutes, stirring occasionally. Sprinkle mixture with flour; cook 1 minute, stirring frequently.

3. Add chicken broth, tomatoes and pepper sauce; bring to a boil over high heat. Reduce heat to medium; simmer, uncovered, 10 minutes or until chicken is no longer pink in center, vegetables are tender and sauce is slightly thickened.

4. Ladle gumbo into 4 shallow bowls; top each with a scoop of rice. Sprinkle with parsley and serve with additional pepper sauce, if desired.

*Makes 4 servings*

**Nutrients per Serving:** Calories: 378 (26% Calories from Fat), Total Fat: 11 g, Saturated Fat: 2 g, Protein: 31 g, Carbohydrate: 39 g, Cholesterol: 69 mg, Sodium: 176 mg, Fiber: 3 g, Sugar: 6 g
**Dietary Exchanges:** 2 Starch/Bread, 3 Lean Meat, 2 Vegetable, ½ Fat

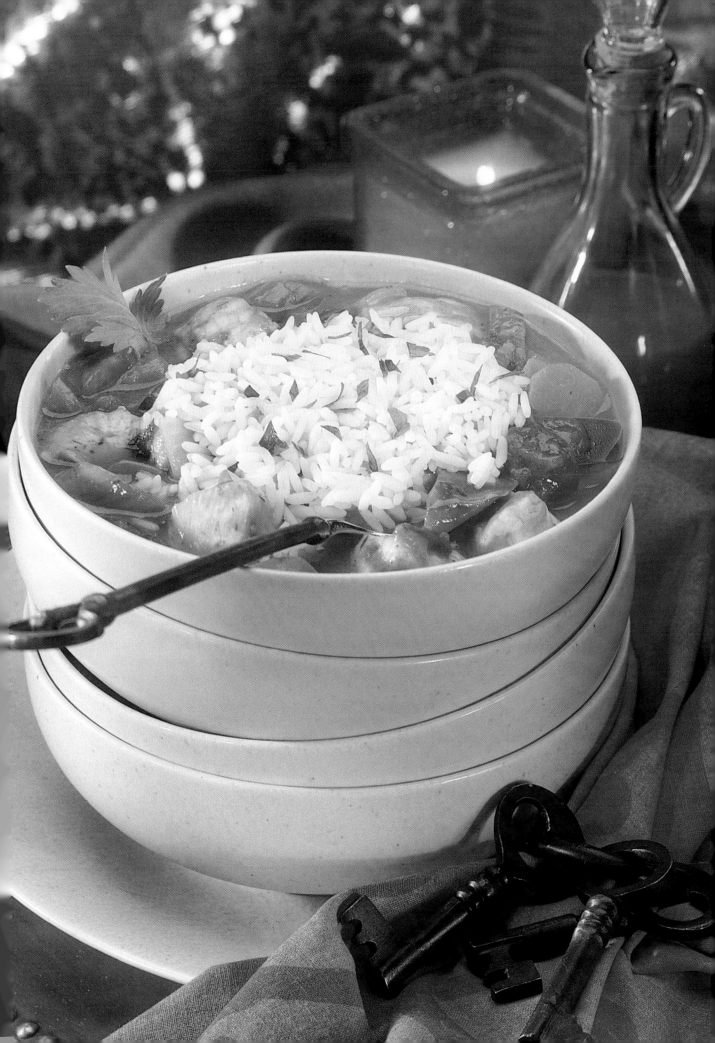

# Fresh Vegetable Lasagna

8 ounces uncooked lasagna noodles
1 package (10 ounces) frozen chopped spinach, thawed and squeezed dry
1 cup shredded carrots
½ cup sliced green onions
½ cup sliced red bell pepper
¼ cup chopped parsley
½ teaspoon black pepper
1½ cups 1% low-fat cottage cheese
1 cup buttermilk
½ cup plain nonfat yogurt
2 egg whites
1 cup sliced mushrooms
1 can (14 ounces) artichoke hearts, drained and chopped
2 cups (8 ounces) shredded part-skim mozzarella cheese
¼ cup grated Parmesan cheese

1. Cook pasta according to package directions, omitting salt. Drain. Rinse under cold water until cool; drain well. Set aside.

2. Preheat oven to 375°F. Combine spinach, carrots, green onions, bell pepper, parsley and black pepper in large bowl. Set aside.

3. Combine cottage cheese, buttermilk, yogurt and egg whites in food processor or blender; process until smooth.

4. Spray 13×9-inch baking pan with nonstick cooking spray. Arrange ⅓ of lasagna noodles in bottom of pan. Spread with half *each* of cottage cheese mixture, spinach mixture, mushrooms, artichokes and mozzarella. Repeat layers, ending with noodles. Sprinkle with Parmesan cheese.

5. Cover and bake 30 minutes. Remove cover; continue baking 20 minutes or until bubbling and heated through. Let stand 10 minutes before serving.

*Makes 8 servings*

**Nutrients per Serving:** Calories: 250 (26% Calories from Fat), Total Fat: 8 g, Saturated Fat: 4 g, Protein: 22 g, Carbohydrate: 26 g, Cholesterol: 22 mg, Sodium: 508 mg, Fiber: 5 g, Sugar: 6 g
**Dietary Exchanges:** 1 Starch/Bread, 2 Lean Meat, 2 Vegetable, ½ Fat

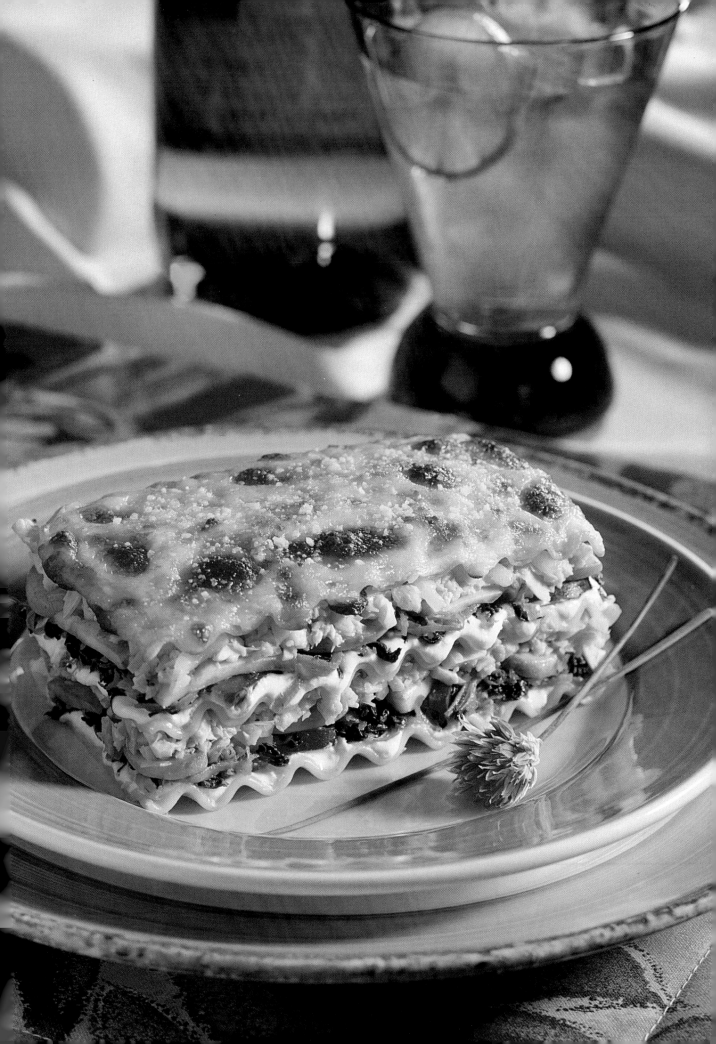

# Beef & Bean Burritos

*Steak plays a supporting role in these easy-to-make burritos. It's the bold flavors of cilantro and green chilies that capture the essence of Mexican cuisine.*

> **Nonstick cooking spray**
> ½ **pound beef top round steak, cut into ½-inch strips**
> 3 **cloves garlic, minced**
> 1 **can (about 15 ounces) pinto beans, rinsed and drained**
> 1 **can (4 ounces) diced mild green chilies, drained**
> ¼ **cup finely chopped cilantro**
> 6 **(6-inch) flour tortillas**
> ½ **cup (2 ounces) shredded reduced-fat Cheddar cheese**
> **Salsa (optional)**
> **Nonfat sour cream (optional)**

1. Spray nonstick skillet with cooking spray; heat over medium heat. Add steak and garlic; cook and stir 5 minutes or to desired doneness.

2. Add beans, chilies and cilantro; cook and stir 5 minutes or until heated through.

3. Spoon steak mixture evenly down center of each tortilla; sprinkle cheese evenly over each tortilla. Fold bottom of each tortilla up over filling, then fold sides over filling. Garnish with salsa and nonfat sour cream, if desired.                                    *Makes 6 servings*

**Nutrients per Serving:** Calories: 278 (22% Calories from Fat), Total Fat: 7 g, Saturated Fat: 2 g, Protein: 19 g, Carbohydrate: 36 g, Cholesterol: 31 mg, Sodium: 956 mg, Fiber: 1 g, Sugar: trace
**Dietary Exchanges:** 2 Starch/Bread, 1½ Lean Meat, 1 Vegetable, ½ Fat

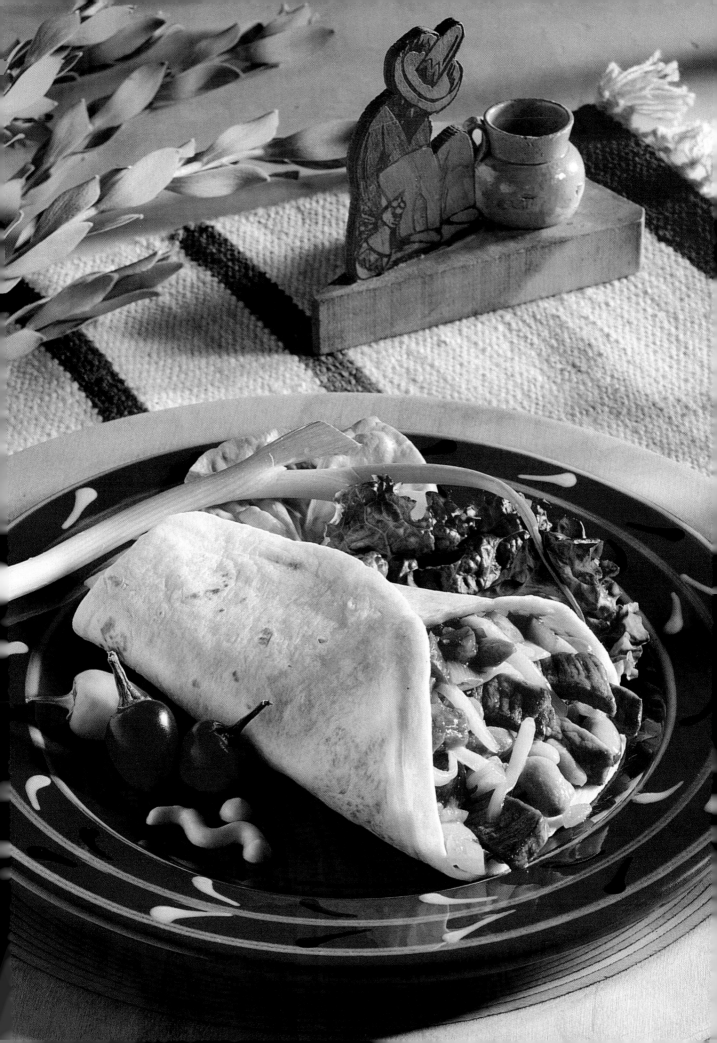

# Desserts

## Apple-Cherry Crisp

**1 pound Granny Smith apples, peeled, cored and sliced ¼ inch thick**
**1 can (16 ounces) tart pie cherries packed in water, drained**
**1 can (16 ounces) dark sweet pitted cherries in heavy syrup, drained**
**2 teaspoons vanilla**
**1 teaspoon cinnamon**
**1 cup fruit-juice-sweetened granola without raisins\***
**⅓ cup sliced almonds**
**1 quart fat-free vanilla ice cream or frozen yogurt**

1. Preheat oven to 350°F. Spray an 11×7-inch glass baking dish with nonstick cooking spray; set aside.

2. Combine apples, cherries, vanilla and cinnamon in large bowl; stir until well blended. Spoon into prepared baking dish. Cover with foil; bake 30 minutes.

3. Remove from oven; stir to distribute juices. Sprinkle granola and almonds evenly over fruit. Bake, uncovered, 15 minutes more or until juice is bubbling and almonds are golden; serve warm or at room temperature topped with ice cream.          *Makes 8 servings*

\*Available in the health food section of supermarkets.

**Nutrients per Serving:** Calories: 296 (15% Calories from Fat), Total Fat: 5 g, Saturated Fat: 2 g, Protein: 7 g, Carbohydrate: 59 g, Cholesterol: 0 mg, Sodium: 100 mg, Fiber: 3 g, Sugar: 28 g
**Dietary Exchanges:** 2 Starch/Bread, 2 Fruit, 1 Fat

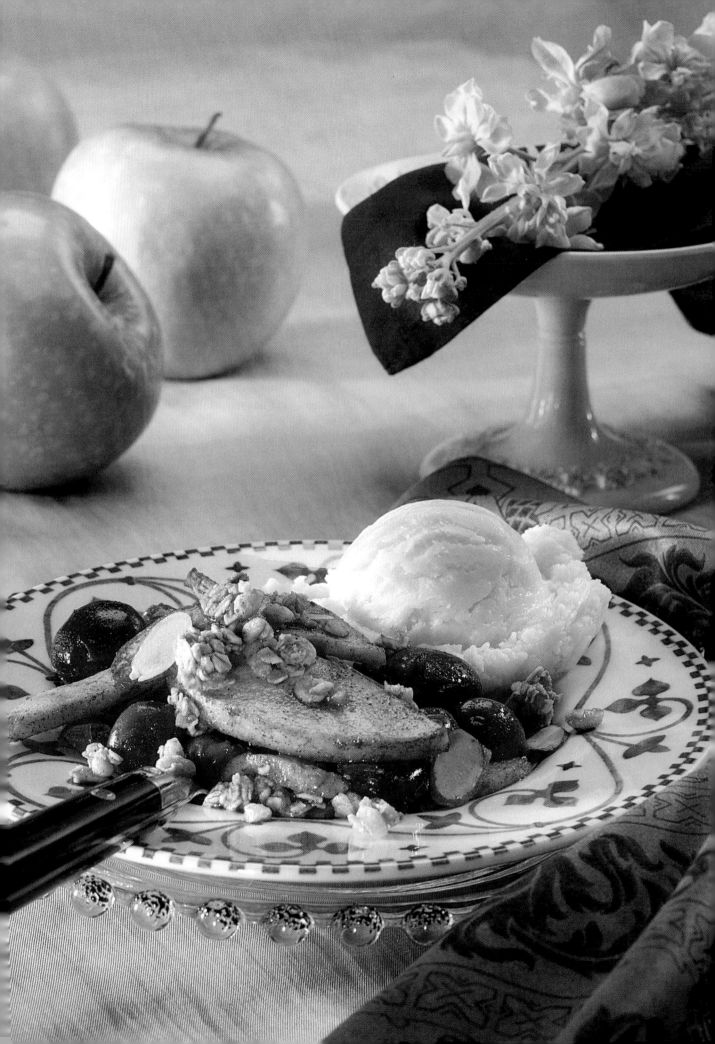

# Mixed Berry Cheesecake

**Crust:**
  1½ cups fruit-juice-sweetened breakfast cereal flakes*
  15 dietetic butter-flavored cookies*
  1 tablespoon vegetable oil

**Cheesecake:**
  2 packages (8 ounces each) fat-free cream cheese, softened
  2 cartons (8 ounces each) nonfat raspberry yogurt
  1 package (8 ounces) Neufchâtel cream cheese, softened
  ½ cup all-fruit seedless blackberry preserves
  ½ cup all-fruit blueberry preserves
  6 packages artificial sweetener *or* equivalent of ¼ cup sugar
  1 tablespoon vanilla
  ¼ cup water
  1 package (0.3 ounce) sugar-free strawberry-flavored gelatin

**Topping:**
  3 cups fresh or frozen unsweetened mixed berries, thawed

*Available in the health food section of supermarkets.

1. Preheat oven to 400°F. Spray 10-inch springform pan with nonstick cooking spray.

2. To prepare crust, combine cereal, cookies and oil in food processor; process with on/off pulses until finely crushed. Press firmly onto bottom and ½ inch up side of pan. Bake 5 to 8 minutes or until crust is golden brown.

3. To prepare cheesecake, combine cream cheese, yogurt, Neufchâtel cheese, preserves, artificial sweetener and vanilla in large bowl. Beat with electric mixer at high speed until smooth.

4. Combine water and gelatin in small microwavable bowl; microwave at HIGH for 30 seconds to 1 minute or until water is boiling and gelatin is dissolved. Cool slightly. Add to cheese mixture; beat an additional 2 to 3 minutes or until well blended. Pour into springform pan; cover and refrigerate at least 24 hours. Top cheesecake with berries before serving.

*Makes 12 servings*

**Nutrients per Serving:** Calories: 248 (25% Calories from Fat), Total Fat: 7 g, Saturated Fat: 3 g, Protein: 10 g, Carbohydrate: 35 g, Cholesterol: 15 mg, Sodium: 386 mg, Fiber: 2 g, Sugar: 6 g
**Dietary Exchanges:** ½ Starch/Bread, 1 Lean Meat, 2 Fruit, ½ Fat

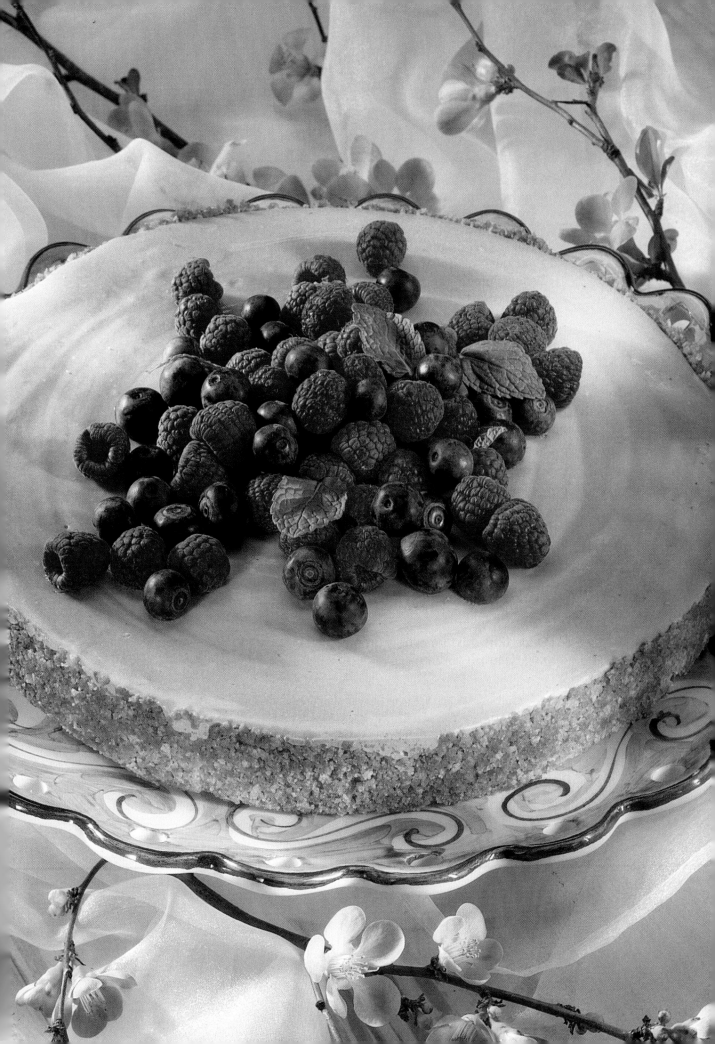

# Key Lime Tarts

¾ cup skim milk
6 tablespoons fresh lime juice
2 tablespoons cornstarch
½ cup cholesterol-free egg substitute
½ cup reduced-fat sour cream
12 packages artificial sweetener *or* equivalent of ½ cup sugar
4 sheets phyllo dough*
Butter-flavored nonstick cooking spray
¾ cup thawed fat-free nondairy whipped topping

1. Whisk together milk, lime juice and cornstarch in medium saucepan. Cook over medium heat 2 to 3 minutes, stirring constantly until thick. Remove from heat.

2. Add egg substitute; whisk constantly for 30 seconds to allow egg substitute to cook. Stir in sour cream and artificial sweetener; cover and refrigerate until cool.

3. Preheat oven to 350°F. Spray 8 (2½-inch) muffin cups with cooking spray; set aside.

4. Place 1 sheet of phyllo dough on cutting board; spray with cooking spray. Top with second sheet of phyllo dough; spray with cooking spray. Top with third sheet of phyllo dough; spray with cooking spray. Top with last sheet; spray with cooking spray.

5. Cut stack of phyllo dough into 8 squares. Gently fit each stacked square into prepared muffin cups; press firmly against bottom and side. Bake 8 to 10 minutes or until golden brown. Carefully remove from muffin cups; cool on wire rack.

6. Divide lime mixture evenly among phyllo cups; top with whipped topping. Garnish with fresh raspberries and lime slices, if desired.

*Makes 8 servings*

*Cover with damp kitchen towel to prevent dough from drying out.

**Nutrients per Serving:** Calories: 82 (17% Calories from Fat), Total Fat: 1 g, Saturated Fat: trace, Protein: 3 g, Carbohydrate: 13 g, Cholesterol: 5 mg, Sodium: 88 mg, Fiber: trace, Sugar: 2 g
**Dietary Exchanges:** 1 Starch/Bread

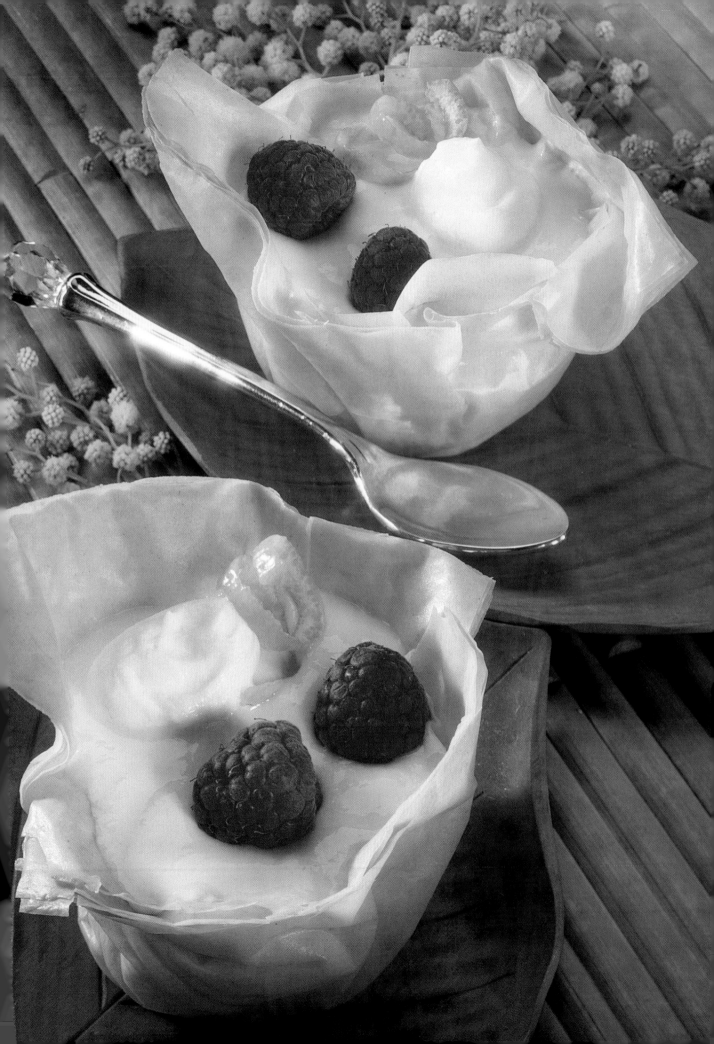

# Chocolate-Strawberry Crêpes

**Crêpes:**
- ⅔ **cup all-purpose flour**
- 2 **tablespoons unsweetened cocoa powder**
- 6 **packages artificial sweetener** *or* **equivalent of** ¼ **cup sugar**
- ¼ **teaspoon salt**
- 1¼ **cups skim milk**
- ½ **cup cholesterol-free egg substitute**
- 1 **tablespoon margarine, melted**
- 1 **teaspoon vanilla**
  **Nonstick cooking spray**

**Filling and Topping:**
- 4 **ounces fat-free cream cheese, softened**
- 1 **package (1.3 ounces) chocolate-fudge-flavored sugar-free instant pudding mix**
- 1½ **cups skim milk**
- ¼ **cup all-fruit strawberry preserves**
- 2 **tablespoons water**
- 2 **cups fresh hulled and quartered strawberries**

1. To prepare crêpes, combine flour, cocoa, artificial sweetener and salt in food processor; process to blend. Add milk, egg substitute, margarine and vanilla; process until smooth. Let stand at room temperature 30 minutes.

2. Spray 7-inch nonstick skillet with cooking spray; heat over medium-high heat. Pour 2 tablespoons crêpe batter into hot pan. Immediately rotate pan back and forth to swirl batter over entire surface of pan. Cook 1 to 2 minutes or until crêpe is brown around edge and top is dry. Carefully turn crêpe with spatula and cook 30 seconds more. Transfer crêpe to waxed paper to cool. Repeat with remaining batter, spraying pan with cooking spray as needed. Separate crêpes with sheets of waxed paper.

3. To prepare chocolate filling, beat cream cheese in medium bowl with electric mixer at high speed until smooth; set aside. Prepare chocolate pudding with skim milk according to package directions. Gradually add pudding to cream cheese mixture; beat at high speed for 3 minutes.

4. To prepare strawberry topping, combine preserves and water in large bowl until smooth. Add strawberries; toss to coat.

5. Spread 2 tablespoons chocolate filling evenly over surface of crêpe; roll tightly. Repeat with remaining crêpes. Place two crêpes on each plate. Spoon ¼ cup strawberry topping over each serving. Serve immediately.

*Makes 8 servings (2 crêpes each)*

**Nutrients per Serving:** Calories: 161 (13% Calories from Fat), Total Fat: 2 g, Saturated Fat: trace, Protein: 8 g, Carbohydrate: 27 g, Cholesterol: 1 mg, Sodium: 374 mg, Fiber: 1 g, Sugar: 6 g
**Dietary Exchanges:** 1 Lean Meat, 2 Fruit

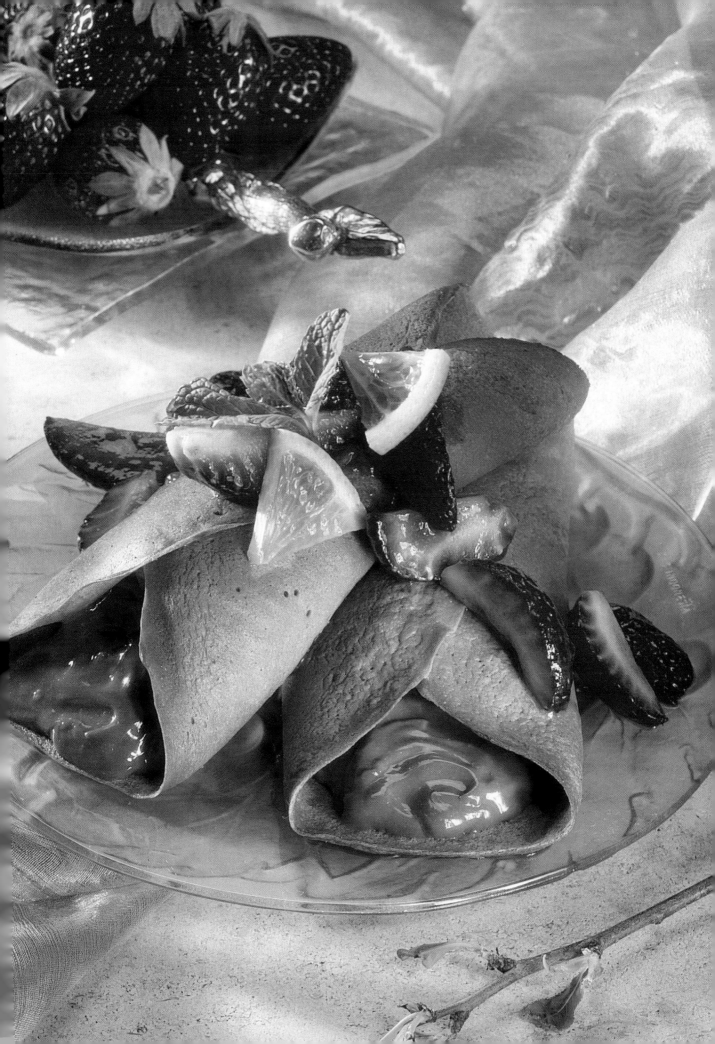

# Lemon Raspberry Tiramisu

*Tiramisu, which literally means "pick me up," is a popular Italian dessert. This variation, which features raspberries rather than coffee and chocolate, is the perfect ending to a special meal.*

**2 packages (8 ounces each) fat-free cream cheese, softened**
**6 packages artificial sweetener *or* equivalent of ¼ cup sugar**
**1 teaspoon vanilla**
**⅓ cup water**
**1 package (0.3 ounce) sugar-free lemon-flavored gelatin**
**2 cups thawed fat-free nondairy whipped topping**
**½ cup all-fruit red raspberry preserves**
**¼ cup water**
**2 tablespoons marsala wine**
**2 packages (3 ounces each) ladyfingers**
**1 pint fresh raspberries or frozen unsweetened raspberries, thawed**

1. Combine cream cheese, artificial sweetener and vanilla in large bowl. Beat with electric mixer at high speed until smooth; set aside.

2. Combine water and gelatin in small microwavable bowl; microwave at HIGH 30 seconds to 1 minute or until water is boiling and gelatin is dissolved. Cool slightly.

3. Add gelatin mixture to cheese mixture; beat 1 minute. Add whipped topping; beat 1 minute more, scraping sides of bowl. Set aside.

4. Whisk together preserves, water and marsala in small bowl until well blended. Reserve 2 tablespoons of preserves mixture; set aside. Spread ⅓ cup of preserves mixture evenly over bottom of 11×7-inch glass baking dish.

5. Split ladyfingers in half; place half in bottom of baking dish. Spread ½ of cheese mixture evenly over ladyfingers; sprinkle 1 cup of raspberries evenly over cheese mixture. Top with remaining ladyfingers; spread remaining preserves mixture over ladyfingers. Top with remaining cheese mixture. Cover; refrigerate for at least 2 hours. Sprinkle with remaining raspberries and drizzle with reserved 2 tablespoons of preserves mixture before serving.                              *Makes 12 servings*

**Nutrients per Serving:** Calories: 158 (9% Calories from Fat), Total Fat: 1 g, Saturated Fat: trace, Protein: 7 g, Carbohydrate: 26 g, Cholesterol: 52 mg, Sodium: 272 mg, Fiber: 1 g, Sugar: 3 g
**Dietary Exchanges:** 2 Starch/Bread

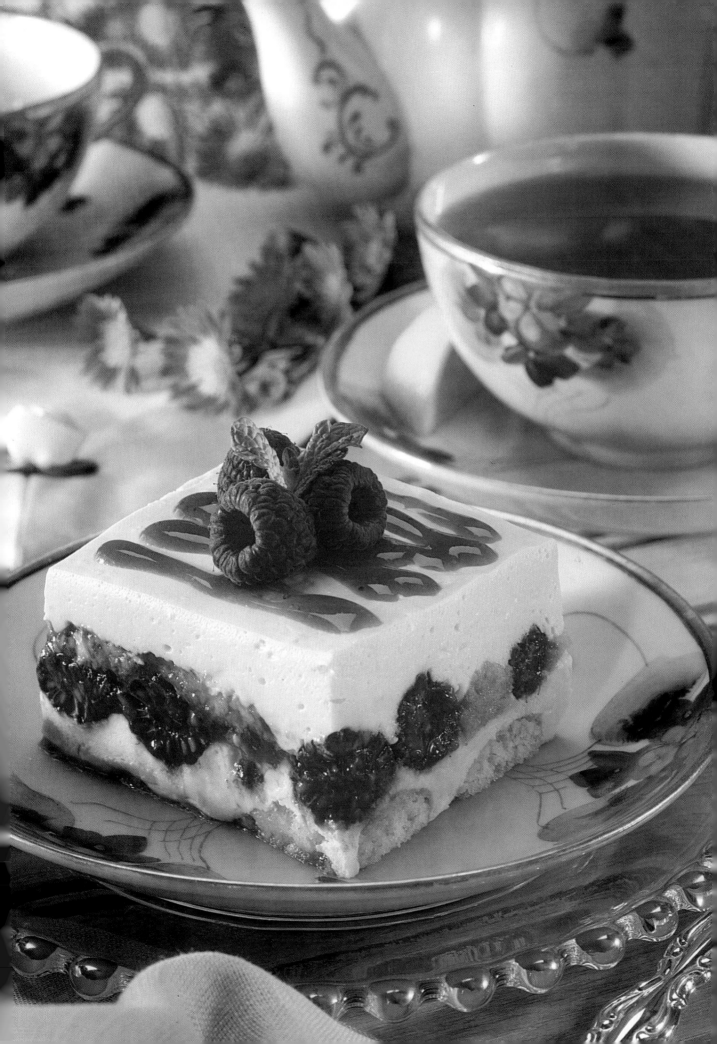

# Tropical Bread Pudding with Piña Colada Sauce

**Bread Pudding:**
   6 cups cubed day-old French bread
   1 cup skim milk
   1 cup frozen orange-pineapple-banana juice concentrate, thawed
   ½ cup cholesterol-free egg substitute
   2 teaspoons vanilla
   ½ teaspoon butter-flavored extract
   1 can (8 ounces) crushed pineapple in juice, undrained
   ½ cup golden raisins

**Piña Colada Sauce:**
   ¾ cup all-fruit pineapple preserves
   ⅓ cup shredded unsweetened coconut, toasted
   1 teaspoon rum *or* ⅛ teaspoon rum extract

1. To prepare bread pudding, preheat oven to 350°F. Spray 11×7-inch glass baking dish with nonstick cooking spray. Place cubed bread in large bowl; set aside.

2. Combine milk, juice concentrate, egg substitute, vanilla and butter-flavored extract in another large bowl; mix until smooth. Drain pineapple; reserve juice. Add milk mixture, pineapple and raisins to bread; gently mix with large spoon. Spoon bread mixture evenly into prepared baking dish and flatten slightly; bake, uncovered, 40 minutes. Cool slightly.

3. To prepare Piña Colada Sauce, add water to reserved pineapple juice to equal ¼ cup. Combine juice, preserves, coconut and rum in microwavable bowl. Microwave at HIGH 2 to 3 minutes or until sauce is hot and bubbling; cool to room temperature.

4. Divide pudding among 8 plates; top each serving with 2 tablespoons of Piña Colada Sauce.                *Makes 8 servings*

**Nutrients per Serving:** Calories: 280 (6% Calories from Fat), Total Fat: 2 g, Saturated Fat: 1 g, Protein: 6 g, Carbohydrate: 61 g, Cholesterol: 1 mg, Sodium: 178 mg, Fiber: 1 g, Sugar: 12 g
**Dietary Exchanges:** 1 Starch/Bread, 3 Fruit, ½ Fat

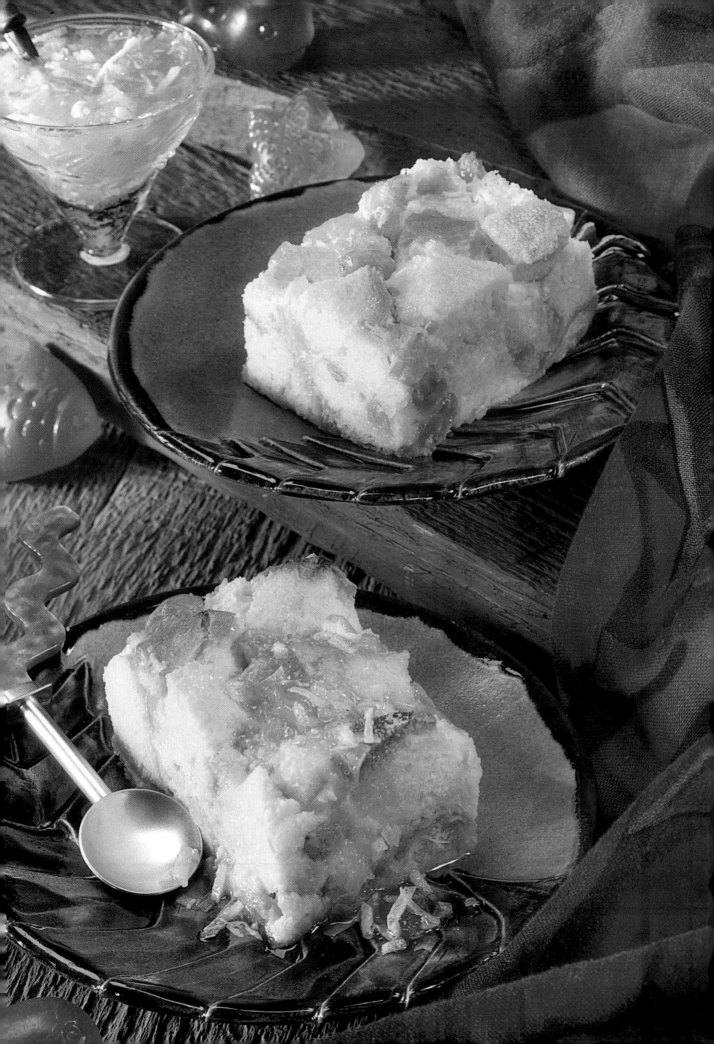

# Sherry-Poached Peaches with Gingered Fruit and Custard Sauce

4 large ripe peaches, peeled, pitted and halved *or* 2 cans (16 ounces each) peach halves packed in juice, drained
⅓ cup dry sherry
1 cup assorted chopped mixed dried or fresh fruit (such as apples, golden raisins, prunes, peaches, apricots, pineapple, raisins and cranberries)
¼ cup water
½ teaspoon fresh minced ginger *or* ¼ teaspoon ground ginger
½ teaspoon grated orange peel
¼ cup all-fruit apricot preserves
1 cup skim milk
½ vanilla bean*
1 egg yolk
3 packages artificial sweetener *or* equivalent of 2 tablespoons of sugar
2½ teaspoons cornstarch

*1½ teaspoons vanilla extract may be substituted for vanilla bean. Stir into cooked custard before serving.

1. Combine peaches and sherry in medium saucepan. Simmer, covered, over low heat for 8 to 15 minutes, stirring often, until peaches are tender. (Cooking time will vary based on ripeness of fruit.) Remove peaches from sherry; cool to room temperature.

2. Combine dried fruit, water, ginger and orange peel in medium microwavable bowl. Cover; microwave at HIGH for 2 to 3 minutes or until fruit is soft. Stir in preserves; cool to room temperature.

3. Pour milk into small saucepan. Cut vanilla bean in half lengthwise; scrape seeds into saucepan. Add bean halves to saucepan. Heat over medium heat just until milk begins to boil; remove from heat. Remove bean halves from milk; discard.

4. Combine egg yolk, artificial sweetener and cornstarch in medium bowl. Beat mixture with wire whisk until thick and lemon colored. Continue whisking mixture while very slowly pouring in hot milk mixture.

5. Slowly pour egg mixture back into saucepan. Cook over medium-low heat, stirring constantly until mixture thickens and coats metal spoon. *Do not boil.* Remove from heat.

6. Divide peach halves and fruit mixture among 4 plates. Top each serving with 2 tablespoons of custard sauce. *Makes 4 servings*

**Nutrients per Serving:** Calories: 290 (5% Calories from Fat), Total Fat: 1 g, Saturated Fat: trace, Protein: 5 g, Carbohydrate: 59 g, Cholesterol: 54 mg, Sodium: 102 mg, Fiber: 4 g, Sugar: 34 g
**Dietary Exchanges:** 4 Fruit

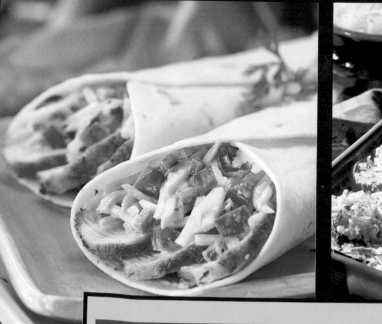

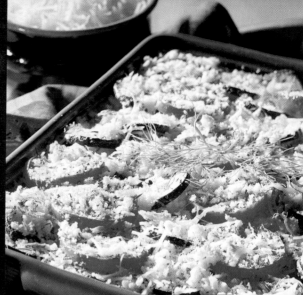

# DIABETIC
# Cooking
## FOR 1 OR 2

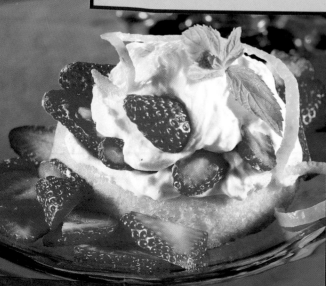

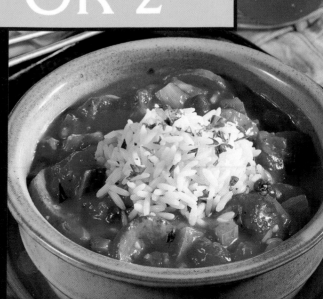

# DIABETIC Cooking FOR 1 OR 2

# Dinner for One or Two

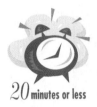

20 minutes or less

*Plain or fancy—you will find the perfect recipe here.*

## Seafood & Vegetable Stir-Fry

2 teaspoons olive oil
½ medium red bell pepper, cut into strips
½ medium onion, cut into small wedges
10 snow peas, trimmed and cut into halves
1 clove garlic, minced
6 ounces frozen cooked medium shrimp, thawed
2 tablespoons stir-fry sauce
1 cup hot cooked rice

*1.* Heat oil in large nonstick skillet over medium-high heat. Add vegetables; stir-fry 4 minutes. Add garlic; stir-fry 1 minute or until vegetables are crisp-tender.

*2.* Add shrimp and stir-fry sauce. Stir-fry just until hot. Serve over rice.              *Makes 2 servings*

**Recipe Tip:** You may substitute ½ cup thawed frozen snow peas for the fresh ones. Add them in step 1 during the last 2 minutes of stir-frying.

Nutrients per Serving: Calories: 279, Calories from Fat: 19%,
Total Fat: 6 g, Saturated Fat: 1 g, Protein: 22 g, Carbohydrate: 33 g,
Cholesterol: 166 mg, Sodium: 724 mg, Dietary Fiber: 2 g

Dietary Exchanges: 2 Vegetable, 1½ Starch, 2 Lean Meat

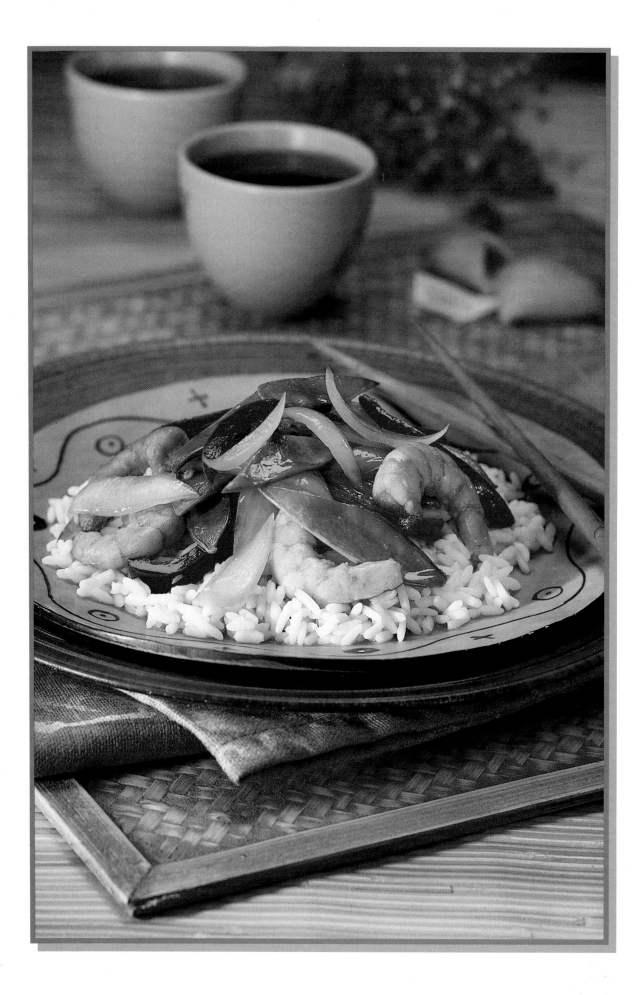

# Chicken & Orzo Soup

Nonstick olive oil
cooking spray
3 ounces boneless
skinless chicken
breast, cut into
bite-size pieces
1 can (about
14 ounces) fat-
free, reduced-
sodium chicken
broth
1 cup water
⅔ cup shredded
carrot
⅓ cup sliced green
onion
¼ cup uncooked
orzo pasta
1 teaspoon grated
fresh ginger
⅛ teaspoon ground
turmeric
2 teaspoons lemon
juice
Black pepper

*1.* Spray medium saucepan with cooking spray. Heat over medium-high heat. Add chicken. Cook and stir 2 to 3 minutes or until no longer pink. Remove from saucepan and set aside.

*2.* In same saucepan combine broth, water, carrot, onion, orzo, ginger and turmeric. Bring to a boil. Reduce heat and simmer, covered, 8 to 10 minutes or until orzo is tender. Stir in chicken and lemon juice; cook until hot. Season to taste with pepper.

*3.* Ladle into serving bowls. Sprinkle with green onions, if desired. *Makes 2 servings*

**Nutrients per Serving:** *Calories: 176, Calories from Fat: 8%, Total Fat: 2 g, Saturated Fat: <1 g, Protein: 18 g, Carbohydrate: 21 g, Cholesterol: 26 mg, Sodium: 182 mg, Dietary Fiber: 2 g*

**Dietary Exchanges:** *1 Vegetable, 1 Starch, 1½ Lean Meat*

---

## *Recipe Tip*

Orzo is a tiny rice-shaped pasta. If it is not available, substitute any very small pasta.

---

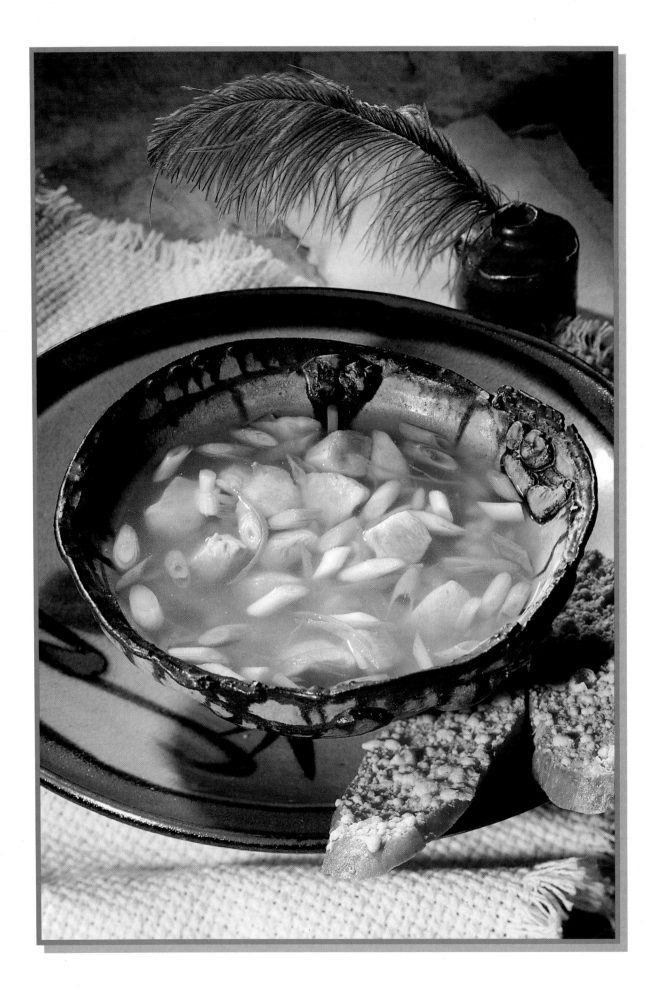

1 tablespoon olive
   oil
½ cup chopped
   onion
¼ cup chopped
   green bell
   pepper
4 ounces low-fat
   smoked
   sausage, cut
   into ¼-inch
   pieces
2 cloves garlic,
   minced
1 cup drained
   canned black
   beans, rinsed
¾ cup undrained
   no-salt-added
   stewed
   tomatoes
1½ teaspoons dried
   oregano leaves
¾ teaspoon ground
   cumin
2 tablespoons
   minced fresh
   parsley
   Hot pepper sauce,
   to taste

# Spicy Black Bean & Sausage Stew

*1.* Heat oil in medium skillet over medium heat. Add onion, bell pepper and sausage. Cook and stir 3 to 4 minutes or until vegetables are tender. Add garlic; cook and stir 1 minute.

*2.* Stir in beans, tomatoes, oregano and cumin, breaking up tomatoes into small chunks with spoon. Bring to a boil; reduce heat to low. Cover and simmer 20 minutes, stirring occasionally. Stir in parsley and pepper sauce.          *Makes 2 servings*

**Serving Suggestion:** Top each serving with a mound of ¼ cup hot cooked rice, if desired. This will add 67 calories and 14 grams carbohydrate to each serving.

*Nutrients per Serving: Calories: 266, Calories from Fat: 30%, Total Fat: 11 g, Saturated Fat: 2 g, Protein: 16 g, Carbohydrate: 39 g, Cholesterol: 26 mg, Sodium: 1022 mg, Dietary Fiber: 10 g*

*Dietary Exchanges: 1 Vegetable, 2 Starch, 2 Fat*

## Recipe Tip

High fiber foods make you feel fuller and are a great way to control hunger. They may also lower total cholesterol and low density lipoprotein (LDL). LDL is often referred to as "bad" cholesterol.

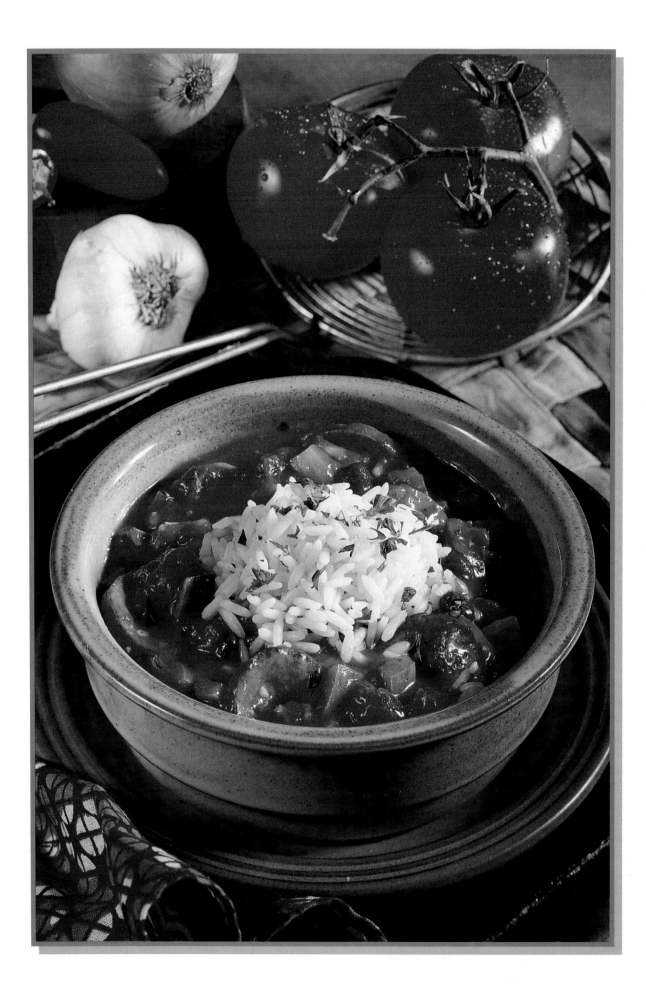

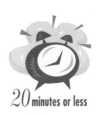

*20* minutes or less

1 reduced-sodium
  bacon slice, cut
  crosswise into
  thirds
3 sea scallops
  (2 ounces)
2 ounces uncooked
  angel hair pasta
1 tablespoon
  reduced-fat
  margarine
2 green onions with
  tops, sliced
1 small clove garlic,
  minced
  Black pepper or
  garlic pepper, to
  taste

# Bacon-Wrapped Scallops on Angel Hair Pasta

*1.* Wrap one bacon piece around each scallop; secure with toothpick.

*2.* Cook pasta according to package directions; drain. Return to pan.

*3.* Meanwhile, heat small nonstick skillet over medium heat. Add scallops; cook 2 to 3 minutes on each side or until bacon is crisp and browned and scallops are opaque. Remove scallops from skillet; discard toothpicks. Reduce heat to low.

*4.* Melt margarine in same skillet.* Add onion and garlic; cook and stir 1 minute or until onion is tender. Remove from heat.

*5.* Add onion mixture to pasta; toss lightly. Place on serving plate. Top with scallops. Season with pepper.

*Makes 1 serving*

*\*If there are enough drippings in the skillet after the bacon is cooked, you may not need the margarine for cooking the onion and garlic. Without the margarine calories are 245, total fat is 4 grams and percentage of calories from fat is 15.*

Nutrients per Serving: *Calories: 305, Calories from Fat: 32%, Total Fat: 11 g, Saturated Fat: 2 g, Protein: 20 g, Carbohydrate: 32 g, Cholesterol: 93 mg, Sodium: 328 mg, Dietary Fiber: 2 g*

Dietary Exchanges: *2 Starch, 2 Lean Meat, 1 Fat*

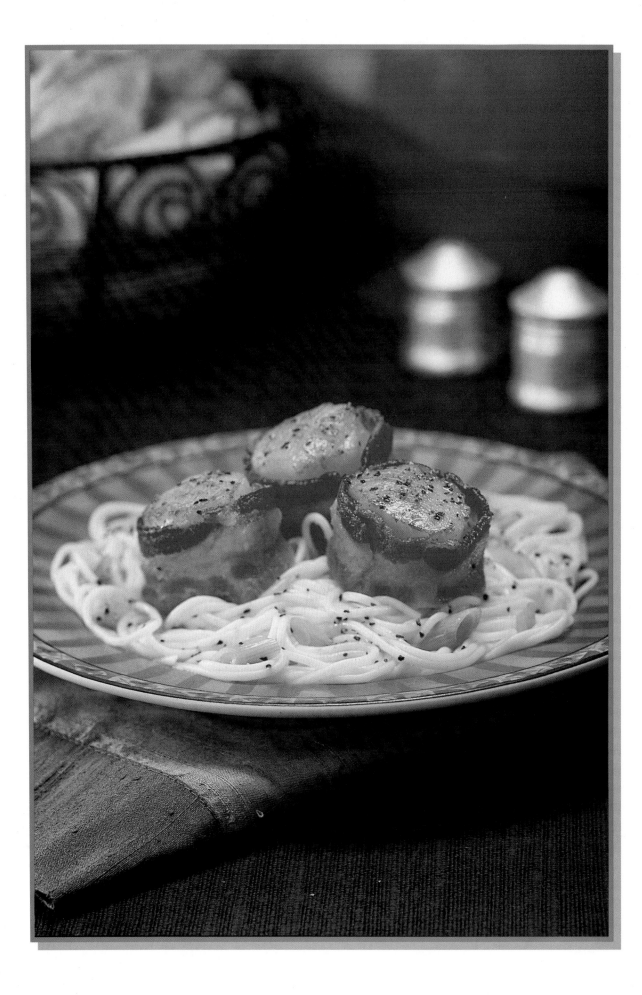

# Curried Chicken Pot Pies

1 tablespoon canola
    oil
¾ cup chopped
    peeled Granny
    Smith apple
⅓ cup thinly sliced
    carrot
¼ cup chopped
    onion
1 clove garlic,
    minced
1 tablespoon
    all-purpose flour
½ teaspoon curry
    powder
⅛ teaspoon salt
⅛ teaspoon black
    pepper
    Pinch ground
    cloves
¾ cup water
1 cup chopped
    cooked chicken
    breast
½ cup no-salt-added
    diced tomatoes,
    undrained
2 tablespoons
    minced fresh
    cilantro
4 refrigerated soft
    breadsticks
    (⅔ of 7-ounce
    package)
    Additional minced
    fresh cilantro
    (optional)

*1.* Preheat oven to 375°F. Spray two 1½-cup casseroles or ovenproof bowls with nonstick cooking spray.

*2.* Heat oil in medium skillet over medium-high heat. Add apple, carrot, onion and garlic. Cook and stir 3 to 4 minutes or until apple and onion are tender. Add flour, curry powder, salt, pepper and cloves. Cook and stir over medium heat 1 minute. Stir in water. Cook, stirring constantly, until liquid boils and thickens. Stir in chicken and tomatoes. Cook 3 to 4 minutes or until heated through. Stir in 2 tablespoons cilantro. Spoon into prepared casseroles.

*3.* Arrange 2 breadsticks over top of chicken mixture in each bowl. Sprinkle additional cilantro over tops, if desired.

*4.* Bake 15 to 17 minutes or until breadsticks are browned and filling is bubbly.     *Makes 2 servings*

**Note:** Leftover breadstick dough may be refrigerated in an airtight container and reserved for another use.

Nutrients per Serving: *Calories: 408, Calories from Fat: 27%, Total Fat: 12 g, Saturated Fat: 2 g, Protein: 23 g, Carbohydrate: 48 g, Cholesterol: 44 mg, Sodium: 685 mg, Dietary Fiber: 4 g*

**Dietary Exchanges:** *1 Vegetable, ½ Fruit, 2½ Starch, 2 Lean Meat, 1 Fat*

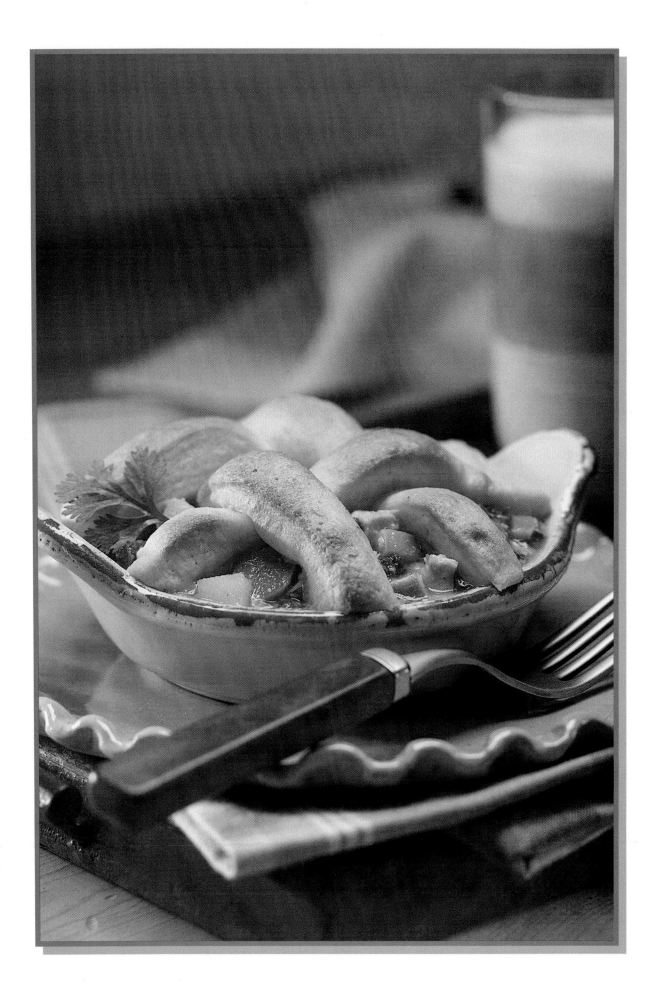

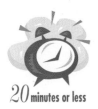

**20** minutes or less

CARB

# Grilled Salsa Turkey Burger

3 ounces lean
    ground turkey
1 tablespoon mild
    or medium salsa
1 tablespoon
    crushed baked
    tortilla chips
1 ounce reduced-fat
    Monterey Jack
    cheese slice
    (optional)
1 whole wheat
    hamburger bun,
    split
1 lettuce leaf
    Additional salsa

*1.* Combine turkey, 1 tablespoon salsa and chips in small bowl; mix lightly. Shape into patty. Lightly oil grid or broiler rack to prevent sticking.

*2.* Grill over medium-hot coals or broil 4 to 6 inches from heat 6 minutes on each side or until no longer pink in center, turning once. Top with cheese during last 2 minutes of cooking time, if desired. Place bun, cut sides down, on grill during last 2 minutes of grilling time to toast until lightly browned.

*3.* Cover bottom half of bun with lettuce; top with burger, additional salsa and top half of bun.

*Makes 1 serving*

**Nutrients per Serving:** *Calories: 302, Calories from Fat: 32%, Total Fat: 11 g, Saturated Fat: 3 g, Protein: 22 g, Carbohydrate: 10 g, Cholesterol: 63 mg, Sodium: 494 mg, Dietary Fiber: 2 g*

**Dietary Exchanges:** *2 Starch, 2 Lean Meat, 1 Fat*

## Recipe Tip

When purchasing ground turkey, check the package label to be sure it contains only white meat. Ground turkey with dark meat and skin may be high in fat. Choose turkey that is at least 97% lean.

# Baked Pasta Casserole

1. Preheat oven to 350°F. Cook pasta according to package directions; drain. Return pasta to saucepan.

2. Meanwhile, heat small nonstick skillet over medium-high heat. Add beef, onion, bell pepper and garlic; cook and stir 3 to 4 minutes or until beef is browned and vegetables are crisp-tender. Drain.

3. Add beef mixture, spaghetti sauce and black pepper to pasta in saucepan; mix well. Spoon mixture into 1-quart baking dish. Sprinkle with cheese.

4. Bake 15 minutes or until heated through. Serve with pepperoncini, if desired.     *Makes 2 servings*

**Note:** To make ahead, assemble casserole as directed through step 3. Cover and refrigerate several hours or overnight. When ready to serve, bake, uncovered, in preheated 350°F oven for 30 minutes or until heated through.

*Nutrients per Serving: Calories: 282, Calories from Fat: 23%, Total Fat: 7 g, Saturated Fat: 3 g, Protein: 16 g, Carbohydrate: 37 g, Cholesterol: 31 mg, Sodium: 368 mg, Dietary Fiber: 3 g*

*Dietary Exchanges: 2 Vegetable, 2 Starch, 1 Lean Meat, 1 Fat*

1½ cups (3 ounces) uncooked wagon wheel or rotelle pasta
3 ounces 95% lean ground sirloin
2 tablespoons chopped onion
2 tablespoons chopped green bell pepper
1 clove garlic, minced
½ cup fat-free spaghetti sauce
Black pepper
2 tablespoons shredded Italian-style mozzarella and Parmesan cheese blend
Pepperoncini (optional)

## Recipe Tip

Pepperoncini are slender 2- to 3-inch-long chilies that are usually pickled. They are slightly sweet and moderately hot. Look for them in the Italian section of your supermarket.

# Tilapia & Sweet Corn Baked in Parchment

⅔ cup fresh or frozen corn kernels

¼ cup finely chopped onion

¼ cup finely chopped red bell pepper

2 cloves garlic, minced

1 teaspoon chopped fresh rosemary or ½ teaspoon crushed dried rosemary, divided

½ teaspoon salt, divided

¼ to ½ teaspoon black pepper, divided

2 tilapia fillets (4 ounces each)

1 teaspoon olive oil

1. Preheat oven to 400°F. Cut two 15-inch squares of parchment paper or heavy-duty foil; fold each piece in half diagonally.

2. Combine corn, onion, bell pepper, garlic, ½ teaspoon rosemary, ¼ teaspoon salt and half of black pepper in small bowl. Open parchment paper; spoon half of corn mixture on one side of each piece, spreading out slightly.

3. Arrange fillets on corn mixture. Brush fish with oil; sprinkle with remaining ½ teaspoon rosemary, ¼ teaspoon salt and black pepper.

4. To seal packets, fold other half of parchment over fish and corn. Fold and crimp along edges until completely sealed. Place packets on baking sheet.

5. Bake 15 minutes or until fish is opaque. Place packets on serving plates. Cut open packets; peel back paper.

*Makes 2 servings*

Nutrients per Serving: Calories: 189, Calories from Fat: 21%, Total Fat: 5 g, Saturated Fat: <1 g, Protein: 24 g, Carbohydrate: 15 g, Cholesterol: 0 mg, Sodium: 622 mg, Dietary Fiber: 2 g

Dietary Exchanges: 1 Starch, 3 Lean Meat

## Recipe Tip

For a special flavor, roast corn and red bell pepper on foil-lined baking sheet lightly sprayed with nonstick cooking spray in 450°F oven for 10 to 15 minutes or until slightly brown, stirring once. Then proceed with the recipe as directed above.

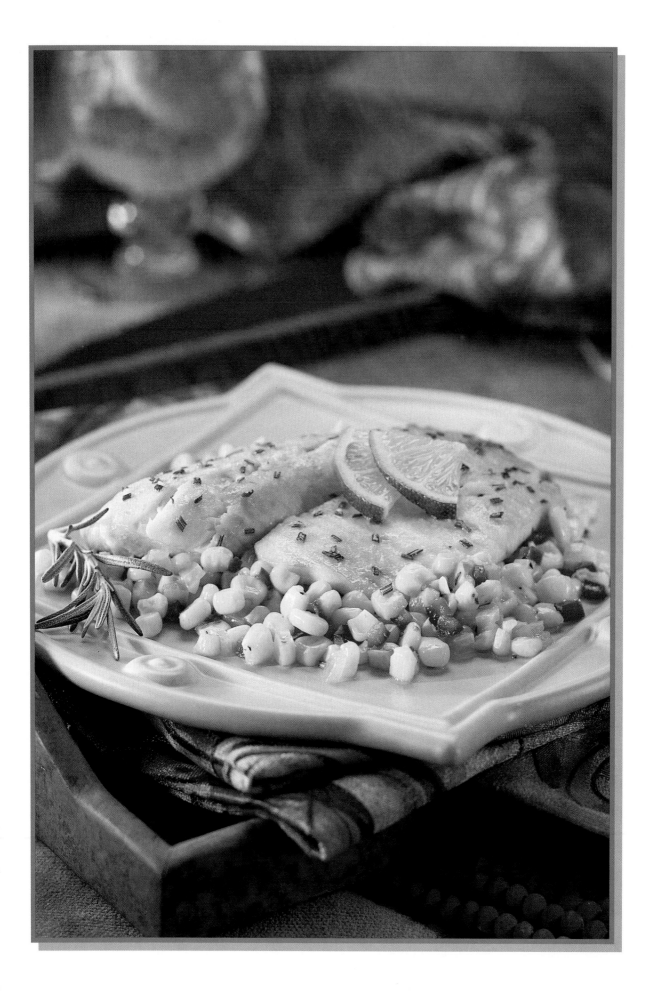

# Crustless Salmon & Broccoli Quiche

¾ cup cholesterol-free egg substitute
¼ cup plain nonfat yogurt
¼ cup chopped green onions with tops
2 teaspoons all-purpose flour
1 teaspoon dried basil leaves
⅛ teaspoon salt
⅛ teaspoon black pepper
¾ cup frozen broccoli florets, thawed and drained
⅓ cup (3 ounces) drained and flaked water-packed boneless skinless canned salmon
2 tablespoons grated fresh Parmesan cheese
1 plum tomato, thinly sliced
¼ cup fresh bread crumbs

*1.* Preheat oven to 375°F. Spray 6-cup rectangular casserole or 9-inch pie plate with nonstick cooking spray.

*2.* Combine egg substitute, yogurt, green onions, flour, basil, salt and pepper in medium bowl until well blended. Stir in broccoli, salmon and Parmesan cheese. Spread evenly in prepared casserole. Top with tomato slices. Sprinkle bread crumbs over top.

*3.* Bake 20 to 25 minutes or until knife inserted into center comes out clean. Let stand 5 minutes before serving. *Makes 2 servings*

**Nutrients per Serving:** *Calories: 227, Calories from Fat: 22%, Total Fat: 6 g, Saturated Fat: 2 g, Protein: 25 g, Carbohydrate: 20 g, Cholesterol: 25 mg, Sodium: 717 mg, Dietary Fiber: 5 g*

**Dietary Exchanges:** *1 Vegetable, 1 Starch, 2 Lean Meat, ½ Fat*

## Recipe Tip

To make fresh bread crumbs, remove the crust from bread slices and tear bread into small pieces. Use any kind of bread, but day-old French and Italian bread make the best bread crumbs.

# Grilled Chicken with Spicy Black Beans & Rice

*1.* Rub chicken with jerk seasonings. Grill over medium-hot coals 8 to 10 minutes or until no longer pink in center.

*2.* Meanwhile, heat oil in medium saucepan or skillet over medium heat. Add bell pepper and chipotle pepper; cook 7 to 8 minutes, stirring frequently, until peppers are soft.

*3.* Add rice, beans, pimiento and olives to saucepan. Cook until hot, about 3 minutes.

*4.* Serve bean mixture with chicken. Top bean mixture with onion and cilantro, if desired. Garnish with lime wedges.

*Makes 2 servings*

Nutrients per Serving: *Calories: 214, Calories from Fat: 18%, Total Fat: 5 g, Saturated Fat: 1 g, Protein: 17 g, Carbohydrate: 30 g, Cholesterol: 34 mg, Sodium: 436 mg, Dietary Fiber: 5 g*

Dietary Exchanges: *2 Starch, 1½ Lean Meat*

1 boneless skinless chicken breast (about 4 ounces)
½ teaspoon jerk seasonings
½ teaspoon olive oil
¼ cup finely diced green bell pepper
2 teaspoons minced dried chipotle peppers
¾ cup hot cooked rice
½ cup canned rinsed and drained black beans
2 tablespoons diced pimiento
1 tablespoon chopped pimiento-stuffed green olives
1 tablespoon chopped onion
1 tablespoon chopped fresh cilantro (optional)
Lime wedges

---

## Recipe Tip

Chipotle peppers are actually dried smoked jalapeño peppers. They have a wrinkled, dark brown skin and a smoky sweet flavor.

# 5 Ingredients or Less

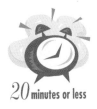

**20 minutes or less**

*You'll be surprised how much flavor five ingredients can bring to a recipe.*

## Ravioli with Tomato Pesto

4 ounces frozen cheese ravioli
1¼ cups coarsely chopped plum tomatoes
¼ cup fresh basil leaves
2 teaspoons pine nuts
2 teaspoons olive oil
¼ teaspoon salt
⅛ teaspoon black pepper
1 tablespoon grated Parmesan cheese

*1.* Cook ravioli according to package directions; drain.

*2.* Meanwhile, combine tomatoes, basil, pine nuts, oil, salt and pepper in food processor. Process using on/off pulsing action just until ingredients are chopped. Serve over ravioli. Top with cheese.

*Makes 2 servings*

**Nutrients per Serving:** *Calories: 175, Calories from Fat: 34%, Total Fat: 10 g, Saturated Fat: 2 g, Protein: 10 g, Carbohydrate: 20 g, Cholesterol: 59 mg, Sodium: 459 mg, Dietary Fiber: 3 g*

**Dietary Exchanges:** *1 Vegetable, 1 Starch, 1 Lean Meat, ½ Fat*

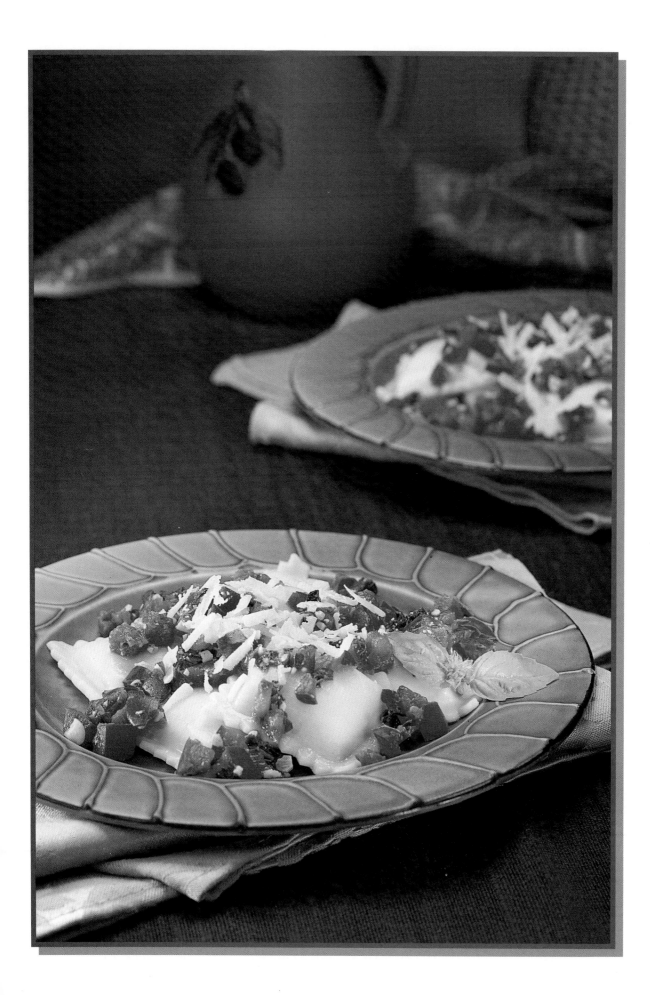

# Grilled Tropical Shrimp

¼ cup barbecue
    sauce
2 tablespoons
    pineapple juice
    or orange juice
10 ounces medium
    shrimp in shells
2 medium firm
    nectarines
6 green onions, cut
    into 2-inch
    lengths, or
    yellow onion
    wedges

*1.* Prepare grill for direct grilling. Stir together barbecue sauce and pineapple juice. Set aside.

*2.* Peel and devein shrimp. Cut each nectarine into 6 wedges. Thread shrimp, nectarines and green onions onto 4 long metal skewers.

*3.* Spray grill grid with nonstick cooking spray. Grill skewers over medium coals 4 to 5 minutes or until shrimp are opaque, turning once and brushing frequently with barbecue sauce.

*Makes 2 servings*

**Nutrients per Serving:** *Calories: 232, Calories from Fat: 7%, Total Fat: 2 g, Saturated Fat: <1 g, Protein: 25 g, Carbohydrate: 30 g, Cholesterol: 217 mg, Sodium: 712 mg, Dietary Fiber: 3 g*

**Dietary Exchanges:** *1½ Fruit, 2½ Lean Meat*

## Recipe Tip

Although shrimp are high in cholesterol, they are naturally low in total fat and saturated fat, making them a good choice for a low-fat diet.

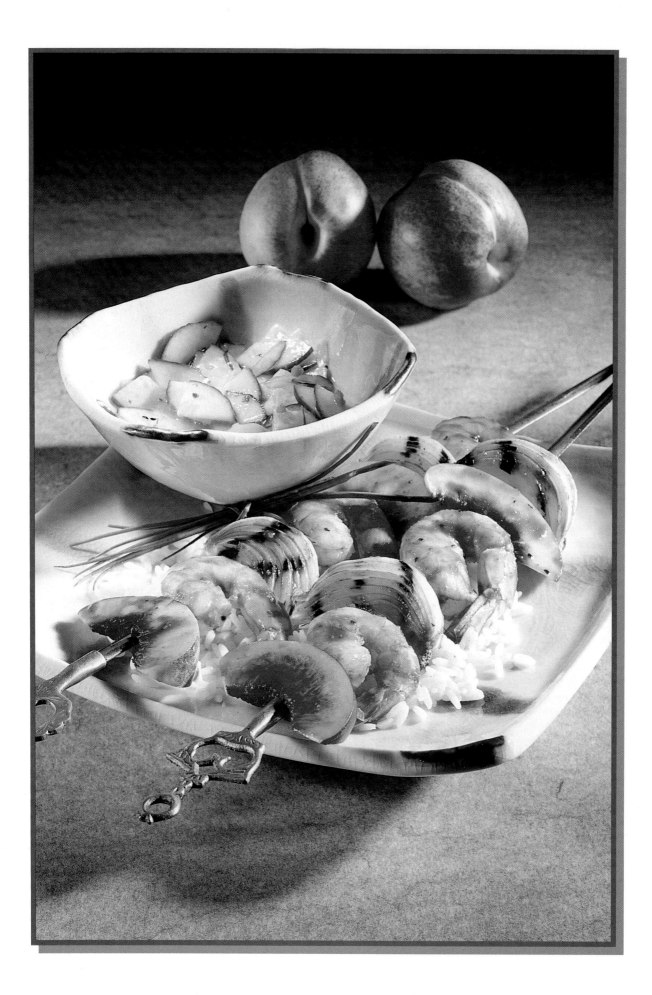

# Spicy Caribbean Pork Medallions

6 ounces pork
  tenderloin
1 teaspoon
  Caribbean jerk
  seasoning
  Nonstick olive oil
  cooking spray
⅓ cup pineapple
  juice
1 teaspoon brown
  mustard
½ teaspoon
  cornstarch

*1.* Cut tenderloin into ½-inch-thick slices. Place each slice between 2 pieces of plastic wrap. Pound to ¼-inch thickness. Rub both sides of pork pieces with jerk seasoning.

*2.* Lightly spray large nonstick skillet with cooking spray. Add pork. Cook over medium heat 2 to 3 minutes or until no longer pink, turning once. Remove from skillet. Keep warm.

*3.* Stir together pineapple juice, mustard and cornstarch until smooth. Add to skillet. Cook and stir over medium heat until mixture comes to a boil and thickens slightly. Spoon over pork.

*Makes 2 servings*

**Nutrients per Serving:** *Calories: 134, Calories from Fat: 23%, Total Fat: 3 g, Saturated Fat: 1 g, Protein: 18 g, Carbohydrate: 7 g, Cholesterol: 49 mg, Sodium: 319 mg, Dietary Fiber: <1 g*

**Dietary Exchanges:** *½ Fruit, 2 Lean Meat*

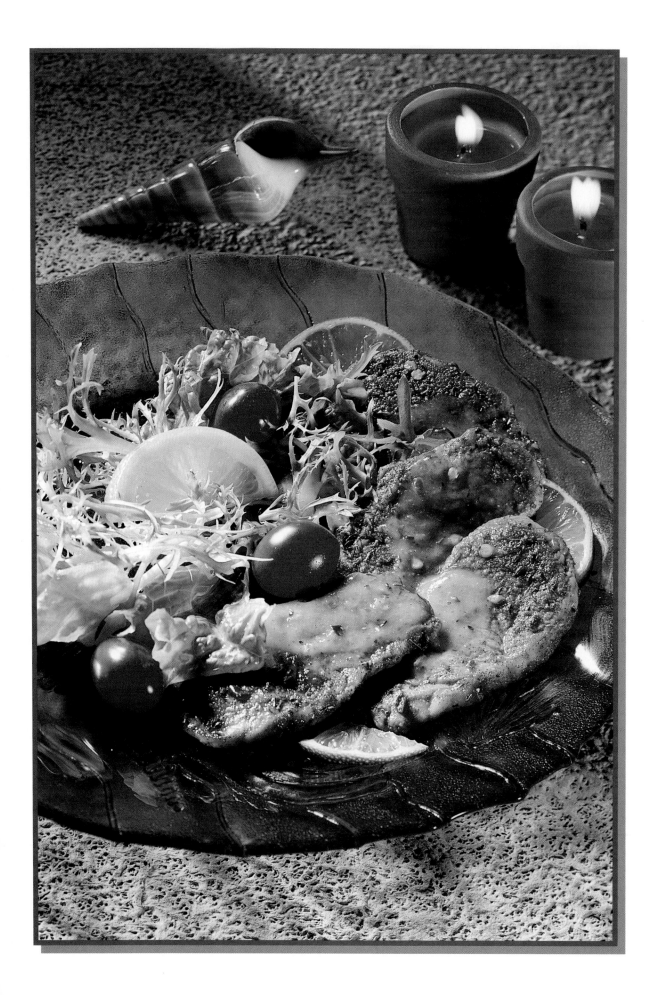

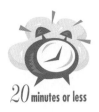

**20 minutes or less**

7 ounces pork
    tenderloin
    Nonstick olive oil
    cooking spray
4 green onions, cut
    into ½-inch
    pieces
2 tablespoons
    hoisin sauce or
    Asian plum
    sauce
1½ cups packaged
    cole slaw mix
4 (8-inch) fat-free
    flour tortillas,
    warmed

# Easy Moo Shu Pork

*1.* Thinly slice pork. Lightly spray large nonstick skillet with cooking spray. Heat over medium-high heat. Add pork and green onions; stir-fry 2 to 3 minutes or until pork is no longer pink. Stir in hoisin sauce. Stir in cole slaw mix.

*2.* Spoon pork mixture onto tortillas. Wrap to enclose. Serve immediately.          *Makes 2 servings*

**Note:** To warm tortillas, stack and wrap loosely in plastic wrap. Microwave on HIGH for 15 to 20 seconds or until hot and pliable.

Nutrients per Serving: *Calories: 293, Calories from Fat: 13%, Total Fat: 4 g, Saturated Fat: 1 g, Protein: 26 g, Carbohydrate: 37 g, Cholesterol: 58 mg, Sodium: 672 mg, Dietary Fiber: 14 g*

**Dietary Exchanges:** *1 Vegetable, 2 Starch, 2 Lean Meat*

## Recipe Tip

When you substitute fat-free flour tortillas for regular ones, you save 3 grams of fat per serving.

# Grilled Portobello Mushroom Sandwich

*1.* Brush mushroom, bell pepper, onion, if desired, and cut sides of bun with some dressing; place vegetables over medium-hot coals. Grill 2 minutes.

*2.* Turn vegetables over; brush with dressing. Grill 2 minutes or until vegetables are tender. Remove bell pepper and onion from grill.

*3.* Place bun halves on grill. Turn mushroom top side up; brush with any remaining dressing and cover with cheese, if desired. Grill 1 minute or until cheese is melted and bun is lightly toasted.

*4.* Cut pepper into strips. Place mushroom on bottom half of bun; top with pepper strips and onion slice. Cover with top half of bun.            *Makes 1 serving*

**Note:** To broil, brush mushroom, bell pepper, onion, if desired, and cut sides of bun with dressing. Place vegetables on greased rack of broiler pan; set bun aside. Broil vegetables 4 to 6 inches from heat 3 minutes; turn over. Brush with dressing. Broil 3 minutes or until vegetables are tender. Place mushroom, top side up, on broiler pan; top with cheese. Place bun, cut sides up, on broiler pan. Broil 1 minute or until cheese is melted and bun is toasted. Assemble sandwich as directed above.

**Nutrients per Serving:** *Calories: 225, Calories from Fat: 22%, Total Fat: 6 g, Saturated Fat: 3 g, Protein: 15 g, Carbohydrate: 30 g, Cholesterol: 27 mg, Sodium: 729 mg, Dietary Fiber: 6 g*

**Dietary Exchanges:** *2 Starch, 1 Lean Meat, ½ Fat*

1 large portobello mushroom cap, cleaned and stem removed
¼ medium green bell pepper, halved
1 thin slice red onion (optional)
1 whole wheat hamburger bun, split
2 tablespoons fat-free Italian dressing
1 (1-ounce) reduced-fat part-skim mozzarella cheese slice, cut in half

# Spiced Turkey with Fruit Salsa

6 ounces turkey breast tenderloin
2 teaspoons lime juice
1 teaspoon mesquite chicken seasoning blend or ground cumin
¼ cup chunky salsa
½ cup frozen pitted sweet cherries, thawed and cut into halves*

*Drained canned sweet cherries may be substituted for frozen cherries.

*1.* Prepare grill for direct grilling. Brush both sides of turkey with lime juice. Sprinkle with mesquite seasoning.

*2.* Grill turkey over medium coals 15 to 20 minutes or until turkey is no longer pink and juices run clear, turning once.

*3.* Meanwhile, stir together salsa and cherries.

*4.* Thinly slice turkey. Spoon salsa mixture over turkey.                    *Makes 2 servings*

**Nutrients per Serving:** *Calories: 125, Calories from Fat: 13%, Total Fat: 2 g, Saturated Fat: 1 g, Protein: 16 g, Carbohydrate: 11 g, Cholesterol: 34 mg, Sodium: 264 mg, Dietary Fiber: 2 g*

**Dietary Exchanges:** *½ Fruit, 2 Lean Meat*

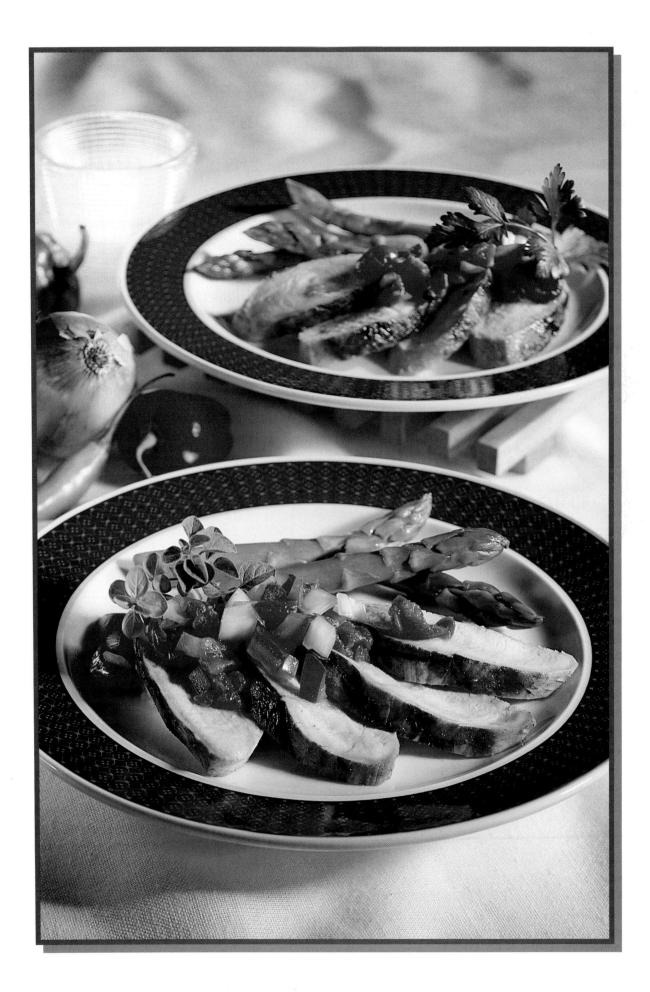

Nonstick olive oil
cooking spray
2 large poblano chili
peppers
½ can (15½ ounces)
black beans,
drained and
rinsed
½ cup cooked brown
rice
⅓ cup chunky salsa
(mild or
medium)
⅓ cup shredded
pepper Jack
cheese or
reduced-fat
Cheddar cheese,
divided

# Black Beans &
# Rice-Stuffed Chilies

*1.* Preheat oven to 375°F. Lightly spray shallow baking pan with cooking spray. Cut thin slice from one side of each pepper; chop pepper slices. In medium saucepan cook peppers in boiling water 6 minutes. Drain and rinse with cold water. Remove and discard seeds and membranes.

*2.* Stir together beans, rice, salsa, chopped pepper and ¼ cup cheese. Spoon into peppers, mounding mixture. Place peppers in prepared pan. Cover with foil. Bake 12 to 15 minutes or until heated through.

*3.* Sprinkle with remaining cheese. Bake 2 minutes more or until cheese melts.          *Makes 2 servings*

**Nutrients per Serving:** *Calories: 289, Calories from Fat: 25%, Total Fat: 8 g, Saturated Fat: 4 g, Protein: 12 g, Carbohydrate: 38 g, Cholesterol: 20 mg, Sodium: 984 mg, Dietary Fiber: 10 g*

**Dietary Exchanges:** *1 Vegetable, 2 Starch, 1½ Fat*

## Recipe Tip

Poblano chilies are dark green medium-sized chilies that range in flavor from mild to quite hot. Anaheim chilies may be substituted if you prefer a mild, sweet flavor.

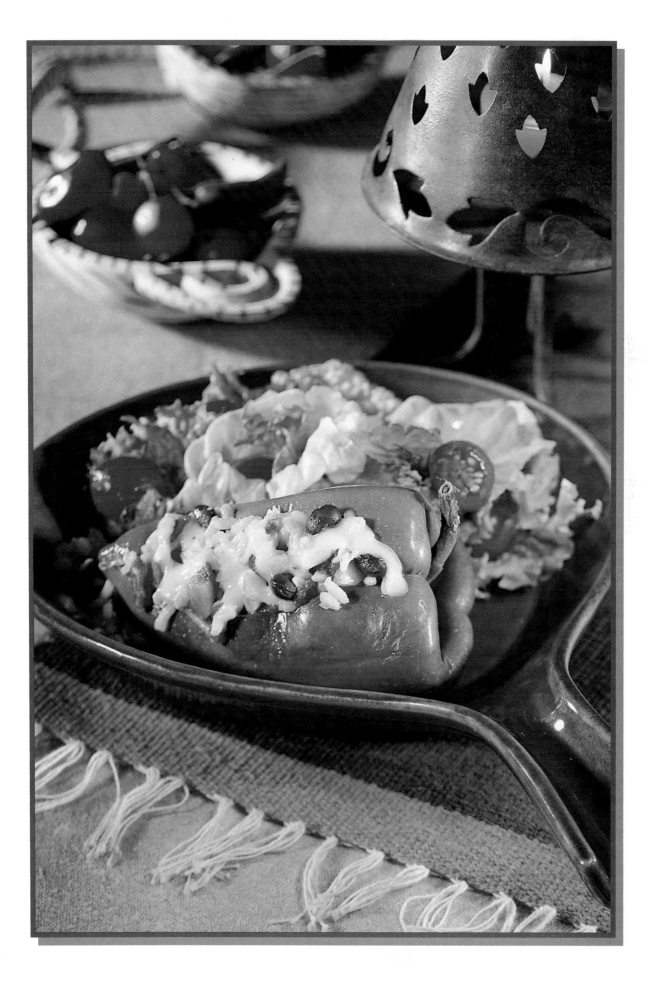

# Grilled Chicken, Rice & Veggies

3 ounces boneless
  skinless chicken
  breast
3 tablespoons
  reduced-fat
  Italian salad
  dressing,
  divided
½ cup fat-free
  reduced-sodium
  chicken broth
¼ cup uncooked rice
½ cup frozen
  broccoli and
  carrot blend,
  thawed

*1.* Place chicken and 1 tablespoon salad dressing in resealable plastic food storage bag. Seal bag; turn to coat. Marinate in refrigerator 1 hour.

*2.* Remove chicken from marinade; discard marinade. Grill chicken over medium-hot coals 8 to 10 minutes or until chicken is no longer pink in center.

*3.* Meanwhile, bring broth to a boil in small saucepan; add rice. Cover; reduce heat and simmer 15 minutes, stirring in vegetables during last 5 minutes of cooking. Remove from heat and stir in remaining 2 tablespoons dressing. Serve with chicken. *Makes 1 serving*

**Nutrients per Serving:** *Calories: 268, Calories from Fat: 23%, Total Fat: 7 g, Saturated Fat: 1 g, Protein: 26 g, Carbohydrate: 25 g, Cholesterol: 54 mg, Sodium: 516 mg, Dietary Fiber: 4 g*

**Dietary Exchanges:** *1 Vegetable, 1½ Starch, 2 Lean Meat*

---

## Recipe Tip

A marinade that has been in contact with raw chicken should only be used as a dipping sauce if it has been brought to a boil and allowed to boil for 5 minutes. This will destroy any salmonella bacteria introduced by the chicken.

---

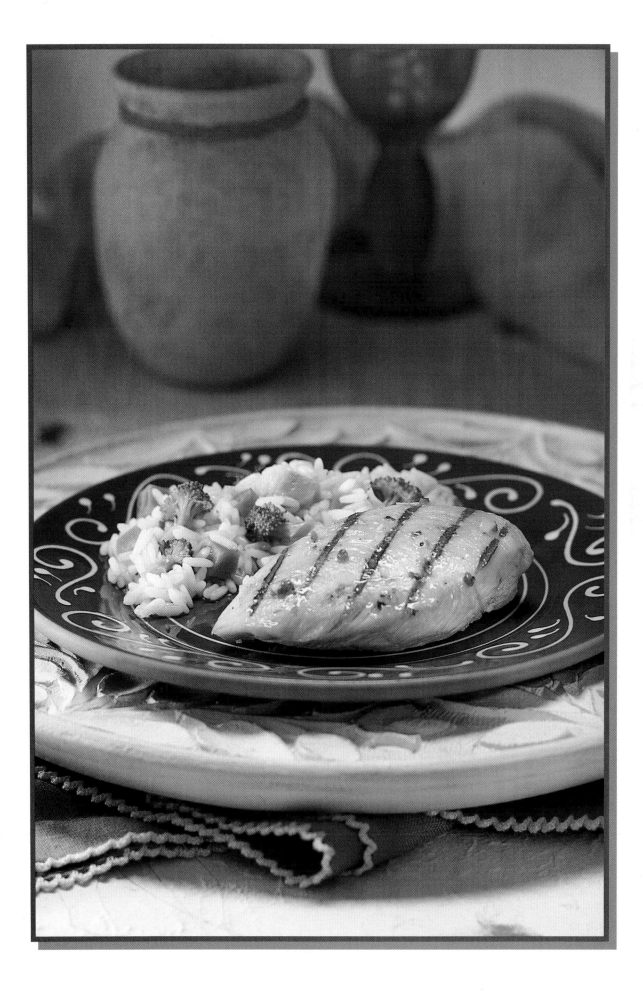

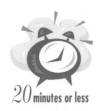

6 ounces beef flank
    steak
½ teaspoon Mexican
    seasoning blend
    or chili powder
⅛ teaspoon salt
    Nonstick olive oil
    cooking spray
4 cups packaged
    mixed salad
    greens
1 can (11 ounces)
    mandarin
    orange sections,
    drained
2 tablespoons green
    taco sauce

# Tex-Mex Flank Steak Salad

*1.* Very thinly slice steak across the grain. Combine beef slices, Mexican seasoning and salt.

*2.* Lightly spray large nonstick skillet with cooking spray. Heat over medium-high heat. Add steak strips. Cook and stir 1 to 2 minutes or to desired doneness.

*3.* Toss together greens and orange sections. Arrange on serving plates. Top with warm steak. Drizzle with taco sauce.          *Makes 2 servings*

**Nutrients per Serving:** *Calories: 240, Calories from Fat: 25%, Total Fat: 7 g, Saturated Fat: 3 g, Protein: 25 g, Carbohydrate: 21 g, Cholesterol: 37 mg, Sodium: 388 mg, Dietary Fiber: 2 g*

**Dietary Exchanges:** *2 Vegetable, 1 Fruit, 2 Lean Meat*

## Recipe Tip

Flank steak is a lean cut of meat,
making it an excellent choice for low-fat cooking.
Cutting it across the grain into very thin strips
helps to tenderize it.

# Chicken & Wild Rice Skillet Dinner

1. Melt margarine in small skillet over medium-high heat. Add chicken; cook and stir 3 to 5 minutes or until no longer pink.

2. Meanwhile, measure ¼ cup of the rice and 1 tablespoon plus ½ teaspoon of the seasoning mix. Reserve remaining rice and seasoning mix for another use.

3. Add rice, seasoning, water and apricots to skillet; mix well. Bring to a boil. Cover and reduce heat to low; simmer 25 minutes or until liquid is absorbed and rice is tender.                     *Makes 1 serving*

**Nutrients per Serving:** *Calories: 314, Calories from Fat: 13%, Total Fat: 5 g, Saturated Fat: 1 g, Protein: 24 g, Carbohydrate: 44 g, Cholesterol: 52 mg, Sodium: 669 mg, Dietary Fiber: 3 g*

**Dietary Exchanges:** *3 Starch, 2 Lean Meat*

1 teaspoon reduced-fat margarine
2 ounces boneless skinless chicken breast, cut into strips
1 package (5 ounces) long-grain and wild rice mix with seasoning
½ cup water
3 dried apricots, cut up

---

## Recipe Tip

Dried apricots are a good source of beta-carotene.

---

# Polenta with Fresh Tomato-Bean Salsa

½ (16-ounce)
      package
      prepared
      polenta
Nonstick cooking
      spray
1⅓ cups chopped
      plum tomatoes
⅔ cup canned black
      beans or red
      kidney beans,
      rinsed and
      drained
2 tablespoons
      chopped fresh
      basil leaves
¼ teaspoon black
      pepper
2 tablespoons
      grated
      Parmesan
      cheese

*1.* Preheat oven to 450°F. Cut polenta into ¼-inch-thick slices. Lightly spray shallow baking pan with cooking spray. Place polenta slices in single layer in baking pan. Lightly spray top of polenta with cooking spray. Bake 15 to 20 minutes or until slightly brown on edges.

*2.* Meanwhile, stir together tomatoes, beans, basil and pepper. Let stand at room temperature 15 minutes to blend flavors.

*3.* Arrange polenta on serving plates. Spoon tomato mixture on top. Sprinkle with cheese.

*Makes 2 servings*

**Nutrients per Serving:** *Calories: 286, Calories from Fat: 17%, Total Fat: 6 g, Saturated Fat: 2 g, Protein: 14 g, Carbohydrate: 48 g, Cholesterol: 9 mg, Sodium: 548 mg, Dietary Fiber: 8 g*

**Dietary Exchanges:** *1 Vegetable, 3 Starch, 1 Fat*

---

## Recipe Tip

Salsa may be cooked, if desired. Cook and stir tomatoes in large skillet over medium heat until hot. Stir in basil and pepper. Serve as directed.

---

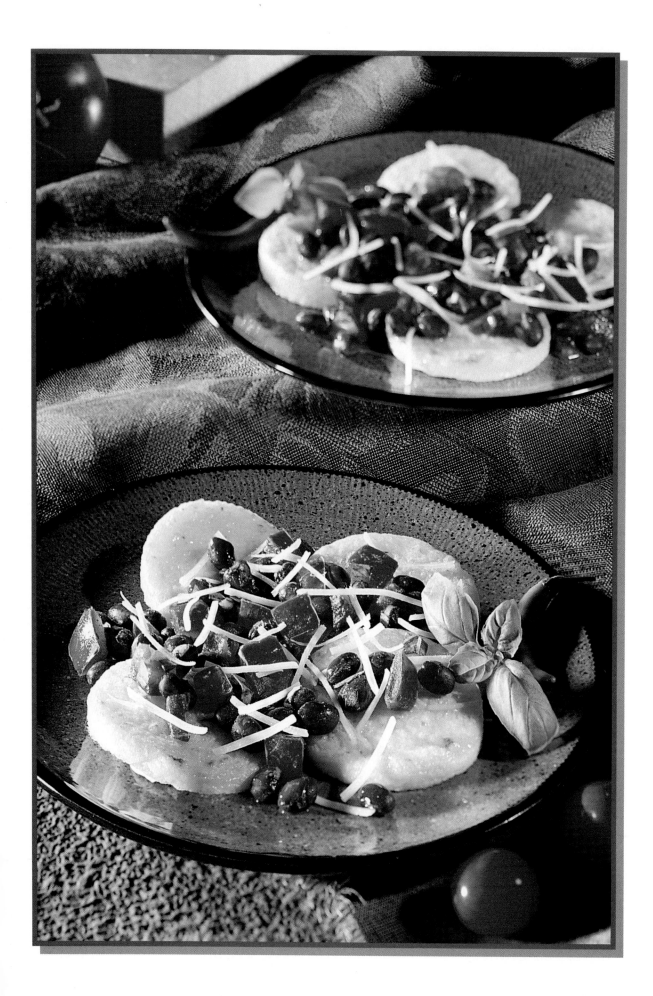

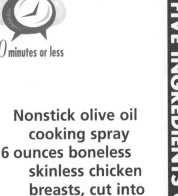

*20 minutes or less*

Nonstick olive oil cooking spray
6 ounces boneless skinless chicken breasts, cut into bite-size pieces
⅓ cup mango chutney
¼ cup water
1 tablespoon Dijon mustard
4 cups packaged mixed salad greens
1 cup chopped peeled mango or papaya
Sliced green onions (optional)

FIVE INGREDIENTS OR LESS

# *Warm Chutney Chicken Salad*

*1.* Spray medium nonstick skillet with cooking spray. Heat over medium-high heat. Add chicken; cook and stir 2 to 3 minutes or until no longer pink. Stir in chutney, water and mustard. Cook and stir just until hot. Cool slightly.

*2.* Toss together salad greens and mango. Arrange on serving plates.

*3.* Spoon chicken mixture onto greens. Garnish with green onions, if desired.          *Makes 2 servings*

**Nutrients per Serving:** *Calories: 277, Calories from Fat: 10%, Total Fat: 3 g, Saturated Fat: 1 g, Protein: 21 g, Carbohydrate: 42 g, Cholesterol: 52 mg, Sodium: 117 mg, Dietary Fiber: 4 g*

**Dietary Exchanges:** *2 Vegetable, 2 Fruit, 2 Lean Meat*

## *Recipe Tip*

Mango chutney is a spicy, chunky condiment most often used as an accompaniment to Indian curries. It ranges in spiciness from mild to hot.

*116*

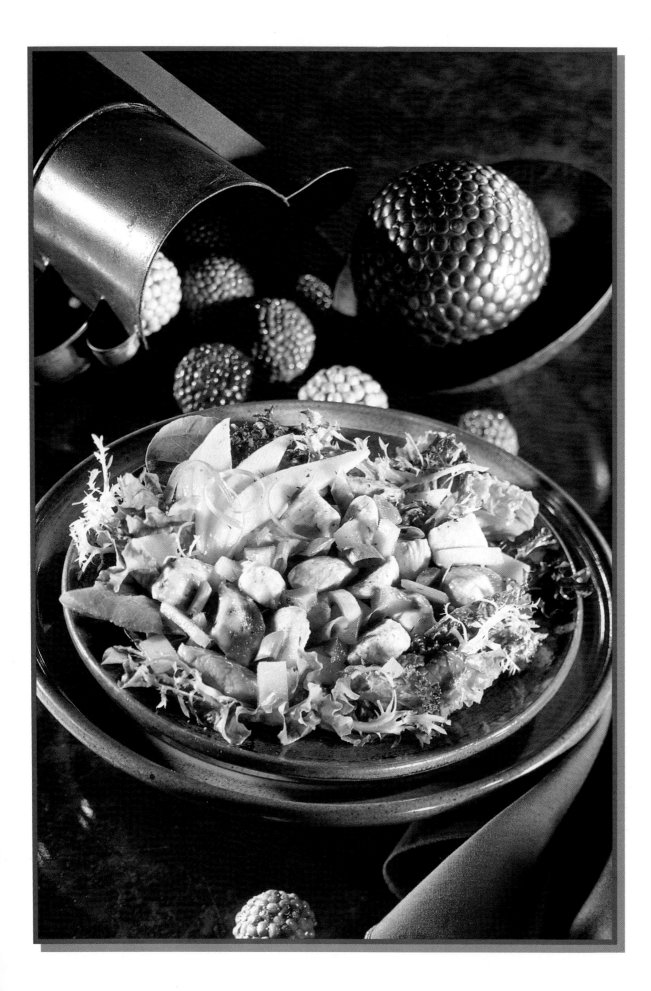

# Two-for-One Dinners

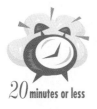

20 minutes or less

*Save part of today's recipe and create something new tomorrow.*

## Jerk Turkey Salad

Reserved turkey from Jamaican Jerk Turkey
   Wraps (page 120)
4 cups packaged mixed salad greens
¾ cup sliced peeled cucumber
⅔ cup chopped fresh pineapple
⅔ cup quartered strawberries or raspberries
½ cup slivered peeled jicama or sliced celery
1 green onion, sliced
¼ cup lime juice
3 tablespoons honey

*1.* Cut reserved turkey into bite-size pieces. Toss together greens, turkey, cucumber, pineapple, strawberries, jicama and green onion.

*2.* Combine lime juice and honey. Toss with greens mixture. Serve immediately.          *Makes 2 servings*

**Nutrients per Serving:** *Calories: 265, Calories from Fat: 6%, Total Fat: 2 g, Saturated Fat: 1 g, Protein: 17 g, Carbohydrate: 48 g, Cholesterol: 34 mg, Sodium: 356 mg, Dietary Fiber: 6 g*

**Dietary Exchanges:** *2 Vegetable, 2 Fruit, 2 Lean Meat*

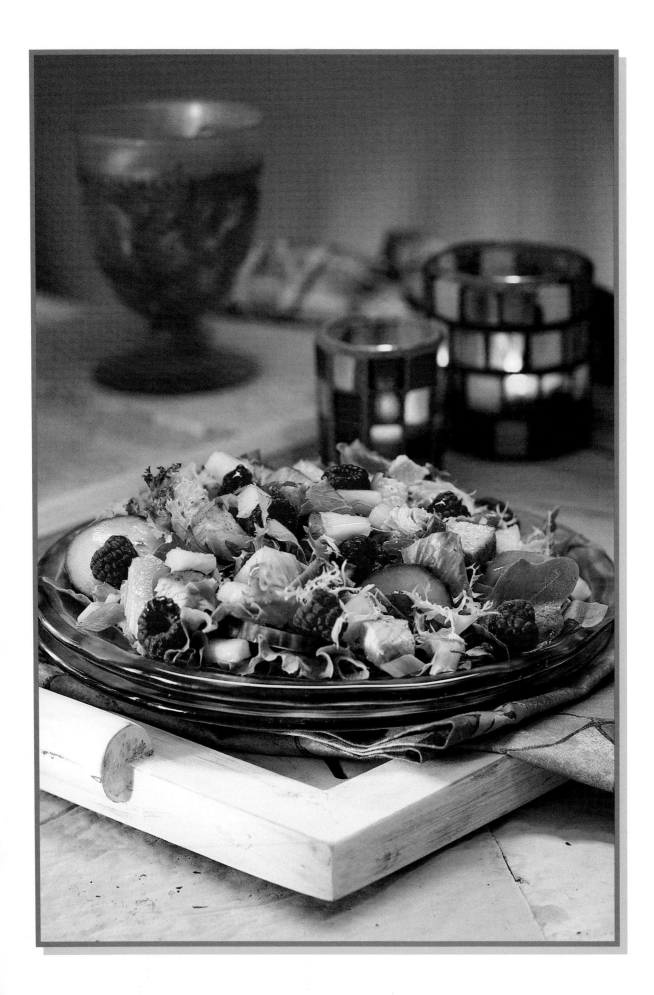

¾ **pound turkey**
   **breast**
   **tenderloin**
**1 tablespoon**
   **Caribbean jerk**
   **seasoning**
**2 cups broccoli slaw**
**1 small tomato,**
   **seeded and**
   **chopped (about**
   **⅔ cup)**
**3 tablespoons**
   **reduced-fat**
   **coleslaw**
   **dressing**
**1 jalapeño pepper,***
   **finely chopped**
**1 tablespoon**
   **mustard**
   **(optional)**
**4 (8-inch) fat-free**
   **flour tortillas,**
   **warmed**

*Jalapeño peppers can sting
and irritate the skin; wear
rubber gloves when handling
peppers and do not touch
eyes. Wash hands after
handling.*

# Jamaican Jerk Turkey Wraps

*1.* Prepare grill for direct grilling. Rub jerk seasoning on both sides of turkey.

*2.* Grill turkey over medium coals 15 to 20 minutes or until turkey is no longer pink and juices run clear, turning once. Thinly slice half of turkey. Cover and refrigerate remaining turkey; reserve for Jerk Turkey Salad (page 118).

*3.* Toss together broccoli slaw, tomato, dressing, jalapeño pepper and mustard. Place sliced turkey on tortillas; spoon broccoli slaw mixture on top. Wrap to enclose. Serve immediately.          *Makes 2 servings*

**Nutrients per Serving:** *Calories: 356, Calories from Fat: 30%, Total Fat: 12 g, Saturated Fat: 2 g, Protein: 20 g, Carbohydrate: 40 g, Cholesterol: 41 mg, Sodium: 1058 mg, Dietary Fiber: 15 g*

**Dietary Exchanges:** *2 Vegetable, 2 Starch, 2 Lean Meat, 1 Fat*

## Recipe Tip

Broccoli slaw, which is slivered broccoli stalks, is now available in most supermarkets. Add it to wraps or pita bread sandwiches, or toss it with coleslaw dressing for a nutritious salad.

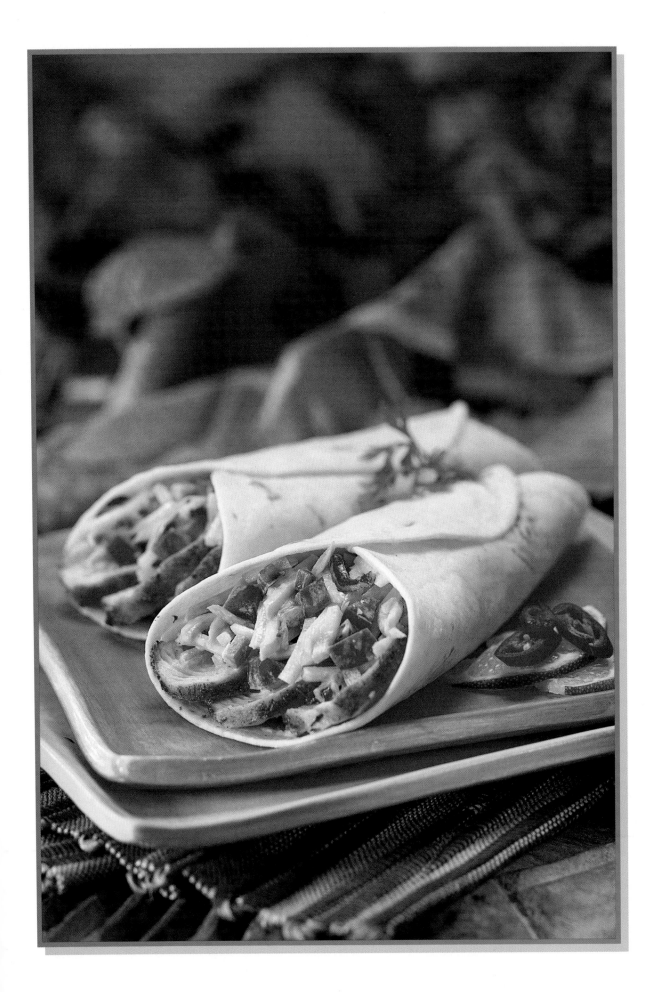

# Thai Curry Stir-Fry

¾ cup fat-free, reduced-sodium chicken broth

1 tablespoon cornstarch

2 teaspoons curry powder

1 tablespoon reduced-sodium soy sauce

¼ teaspoon crushed red pepper

Nonstick olive oil cooking spray

4 green onions, sliced

1 to 2 cloves garlic, minced

3 cups broccoli florets

1 cup sliced carrot

2 teaspoons olive oil

10 ounces boneless skinless chicken breasts, cut into bite-size pieces

⅔ cup hot cooked rice, prepared without salt

1. Stir together broth, cornstarch, curry powder, soy sauce and red pepper. Set aside.

2. Spray nonstick wok or large nonstick skillet with cooking spray. Heat over medium-high heat. Add green onions and garlic; stir-fry 1 minute. Remove from wok.

3. Add broccoli and carrot to wok; stir-fry 2 to 3 minutes or until crisp-tender. Remove from wok.

4. Add oil to hot wok. Add chicken and stir-fry 2 to 3 minutes or until no longer pink. Stir broth mixture. Add to wok. Cook and stir until broth mixture comes to a boil and thickens slightly. Return all vegetables to wok. Heat through.

5. Cover and refrigerate 1½ cups of chicken mixture. Reserve for Curried Chicken & Pasta Salad (page 124).

6. Serve remaining chicken mixture with rice.

*Makes 2 servings*

Nutrients per Serving: Calories: 273, Calories from Fat: 20%, Total Fat: 6 g, Saturated Fat: 1 g, Protein: 28 g, Carbohydrate: 27 g, Cholesterol: 57 mg, Sodium: 308 mg, Dietary Fiber: 5 g

Dietary Exchanges: 2 Vegetable, 1 Starch, 3 Lean Meat

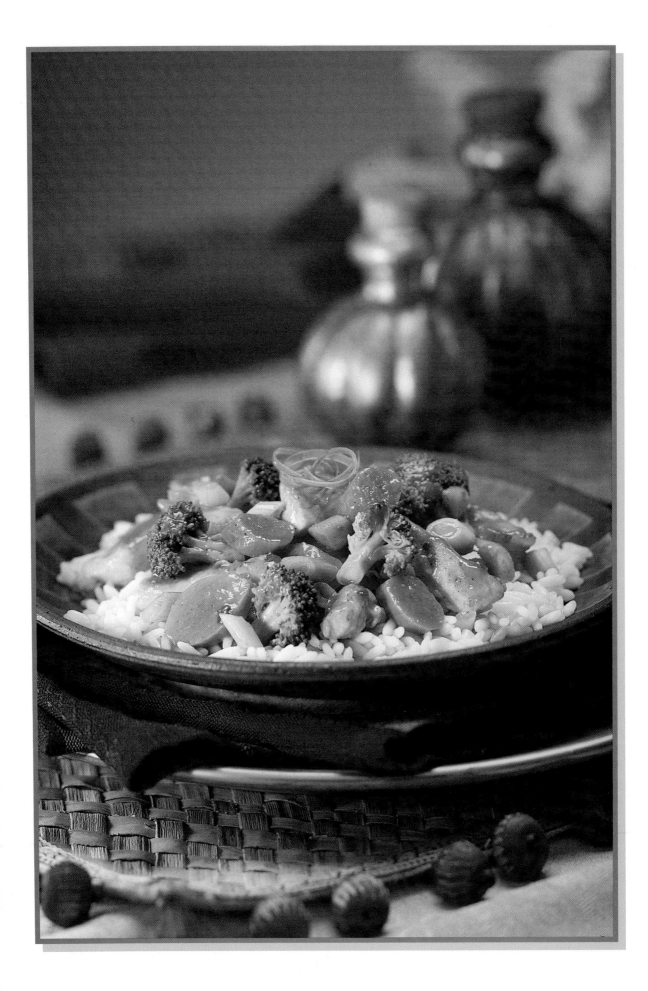

1½ cups reserved
    chicken mixture
    from Thai Curry
    Stir-Fry (page
    122)
⅔ cup cooked small
    shell pasta
½ cup sliced celery
⅓ cup dried
    cranberries or
    tart cherries
¼ cup fat-free honey
    Dijon salad
    dressing
  Salt
2 lettuce leaves

# Curried Chicken & Pasta Salad

*1.* Toss together reserved chicken mixture, pasta, celery, cranberries and salad dressing. Season to taste with salt.

*2.* Cover and refrigerate 1 to 24 hours. Serve on lettuce leaves.                    *Makes 2 servings*

**Nutrients per Serving:** *Calories: 322, Calories from Fat: 11%, Total Fat: 4 g, Saturated Fat: 1 g, Protein: 18 g, Carbohydrate: 55 g, Cholesterol: 29 mg, Sodium: 517 mg, Dietary Fiber: 5 g*

**Dietary Exchanges:** *2 Vegetable, 3 Starch, 1 Lean Meat*

---

## Recipe Tip

Skinless, well-trimmed chicken or turkey breast is lower in fat than all meat products, making it an excellent choice for a low-fat diet.

---

# Pork, Mushrooms, Onion & Pepper

*1.* Sprinkle both sides of pork chops with salt and garlic pepper. Coat large nonstick skillet with cooking spray; heat over medium-low heat. Cook pork 1 to 2 minutes per side side or until brown and barely pink in center. Remove from skillet. Cover and refrigerate half the pork; reserve for Pork & Vegetable Wraps (page 126). Keep remaining pork warm.

*2.* Heat oil over medium heat in same nonstick skillet. Add mushrooms, onion, bell pepper, garlic and salt. Cook 8 to 10 minutes or until vegetables are soft. Add wine, a little at a time, stirring to remove any browned bits from bottom of skillet. Bring to a boil; boil 2 minutes. Serve vegetable mixture over pork chops.                *Makes 2 servings*

**Nutrients per Serving:** *Calories: 264, Calories from Fat: 34%, Total Fat: 10 g, Saturated Fat: 3 g, Protein: 22 g, Carbohydrate: 18 g, Cholesterol: 40 mg, Sodium: 340 mg, Dietary Fiber: 4 g*

**Dietary Exchanges:** *3 Vegetable, 3 Starch, ½ Fat*

1 pound boneless thin-cut pork loin chops
⅛ teaspoon salt
¼ teaspoon garlic pepper
Nonstick cooking spray
1 teaspoon olive oil
1½ cups thinly sliced mushrooms
1 cup diced onion
1 cup diced red bell pepper
1 clove garlic, minced
⅛ teaspoon salt
¼ cup red wine

---

## Recipe Tip

Wine adds a lot of flavor to recipes. Just be sure that wine mixtures cook for 2 or 3 minutes to burn off the alcohol and allow flavors to blend.

---

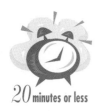

8 ounces reserved
   cooked boneless
   thin-cut pork
   chops from
   Pork,
   Mushrooms,
   Onion & Pepper
   (page 125)
1 tablespoon
   reduced-fat
   mayonnaise
2 teaspoons Dijon
   mustard
4 (8-inch) fat-free
   flour tortillas
1 cup torn spinach
   leaves
½ peeled cucumber,
   diced
1 medium tomato,
   chopped
   Black pepper to
   taste
   Celery salt
   (optional)

# Pork & Vegetable Wraps

*1.* Cut pork chops into strips. Combine mayonnaise and mustard in small cup. Spread on one side of each tortilla. Top with remaining ingredients, seasoning to taste with pepper and celery salt, if desired.

*2.* Fold in 2 sides of tortilla and roll up to enclose filling. Lay seam side down and cut in half. Serve immediately.     *Makes 2 servings*

**Nutrients per Serving:** *Calories: 327, Calories from Fat: 30%, Total Fat: 11 g, Saturated Fat: 3 g, Protein: 24 g, Carbohydrate: 33 g, Cholesterol: 40 mg, Sodium: 637 mg, Dietary Fiber: 14 g*

**Dietary Exchanges:** *3 Vegetable, 1 Starch, 3 Lean Meat, ½ Fat*

## *Recipe Tip*

The mayonnaise-mustard mixture in this recipe may be served on the side as a dipping sauce rather than spread on the tortillas, if desired.

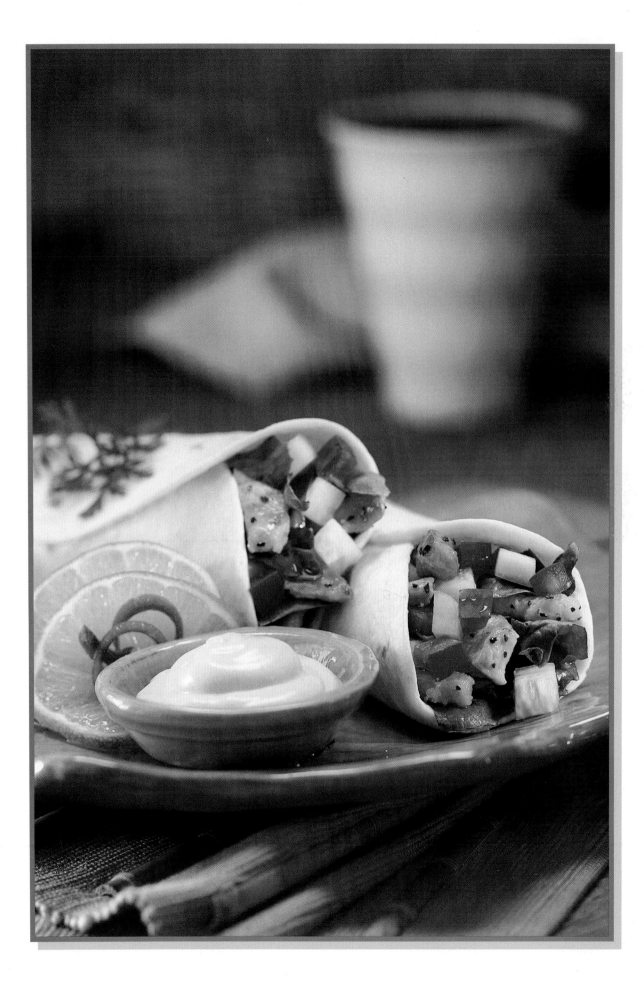

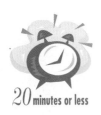

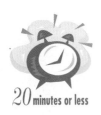 *20 minutes or less*

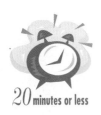 12 ounces ground
sirloin
½ cup chopped
onion
2 cloves garlic,
minced
1 can (8 ounces)
tomato sauce
⅓ cup chopped
carrot
¼ cup water
2 tablespoons red
wine
1 teaspoon dried
Italian
seasoning
1½ cups hot cooked
penne pasta
Chopped fresh
parsley

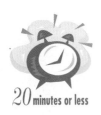 **TWO-FOR-ONE DINNERS**

# Bolognese Sauce & Penne Pasta

*1.* Heat medium saucepan over medium heat until hot. Add beef, onion and garlic; cook and stir 5 to 7 minutes, breaking up meat with spoon, until beef is browned. Remove ½ cup of beef mixture and refrigerate; reserve for Speedy Tacos (page 129).

*2.* To beef mixture remaining in saucepan, add tomato sauce, carrot, water, wine and Italian seasoning. Bring to a boil. Reduce heat and simmer 15 minutes. Place pasta in bowls and top with sauce. Sprinkle with parsley.                    *Makes 2 servings*

**Nutrients per Serving:** *Calories: 292, Calories from Fat: 14%, Total Fat: 5 g, Saturated Fat: 2 g, Protein: 21 g, Carbohydrate: 40 g, Cholesterol: 45 mg, Sodium: 734 mg, Dietary Fiber: 4 g*

**Dietary Exchanges:** *1 Vegetable, 2 Starch, 2 Lean Meat*

---

## Recipe Tip

Carrots add sweetness that reduces the acidic flavor of this quick bolognese sauce.

---

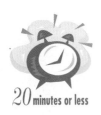 128

# Speedy Tacos

*20* minutes or less

*1.* In small saucepan, heat beef, tomato sauce and seasonings until hot.

*2.* Warm taco shells in oven following package directions.

*3.* Fill taco shells with meat mixture, cheese, lettuce, tomato and onion. Serve with pepper sauce, if desired.                              *Makes 2 servings*

**Nutrients per Serving** *(3 tacos):  Calories: 342, Calories from Fat: 36%, Total Fat: 14 g, Saturated Fat: 4 g, Protein: 19 g, Carbohydrate: 36 g, Cholesterol: 40 mg, Sodium: 706 mg, Dietary Fiber: 5 g*

**Dietary Exchanges:** *1 Vegetable, 2 Starch, 2 Lean Meat, 1½ Fat*

---

### Recipe Tip

If you wish to reduce the fat in these easy tacos, simply divide the filling among 4 taco shells instead of 6.

---

½ cup reserved cooked beef mixture from Bolognese Sauce & Penne Pasta (page 128)
⅓ cup no-salt-added tomato sauce
1 tablespoon taco seasonings
6 taco shells
¼ cup (2 ounces) shredded reduced-fat Cheddar cheese
½ cup shredded lettuce
⅓ cup diced tomato
¼ cup chopped onion
Hot pepper sauce (optional)

**4 ears fresh corn,
   unhusked**
**1 (12-ounce) salmon
   fillet, cut into
   4 pieces**
**2 tablespoons plus
   1 teaspoon
   fresh lime juice,
   divided**
**1 clove garlic,
   minced**
**1 teaspoon chili
   powder**
**½ teaspoon ground
   cumin**
**½ teaspoon oregano
   leaves**
**¼ teaspoon salt,
   divided**
**⅛ teaspoon black
   pepper**
**2 teaspoons
   margarine,
   melted**
**2 teaspoons minced
   fresh cilantro**

# Southwest Roasted Salmon & Corn

*1.* Preheat oven to 400°F. Spray shallow 1-quart baking dish with nonstick cooking spray. Pull back husks from each ear of corn, leaving husks attached. Discard silk. Soak ears in cold water 20 minutes.

*2.* Place salmon, skin sides down, in prepared baking dish. Pour 2 tablespoons lime juice over fillets. Marinate at room temperature 15 minutes.

*3.* Combine garlic, chili powder, cumin, oregano, ⅛ teaspoon salt and pepper in small bowl. Pat salmon lightly with paper towel to dry. Rub garlic mixture on tops and sides of salmon.

*4.* Remove corn from water; pat kernels dry with paper towels. Bring husks back up over each ear; secure at top with thin strips of corn husk. Place corn on 1 side of oven rack. Roast 10 minutes. Turn over with tongs.

*5.* Place salmon on other side of oven rack. Roast 15 minutes or until salmon is opaque and flakes when tested with fork, and corn is tender.

*6.* Combine margarine, cilantro and remaining ⅛ teaspoon salt in small bowl. Remove husks from corn. Brush over two ears of corn.

*7.* Set aside two ears of corn and two pieces of salmon. Wrap and refrigerate. Reserve for Salmon, Corn & Barley Chowder (page 132). Serve remaining seasoned corn and salmon.    *Makes 2 servings*

**Nutrients per Serving:** *Calories: 186, Calories from Fat: 29%, Total Fat: 6 g, Saturated Fat: 1 g, Protein: 19 g, Carbohydrate: 16 g, Cholesterol: 43 mg, Sodium: 243 mg, Dietary Fiber: 2 g*

**Dietary Exchanges:** *1 Starch, 1 Lean Meat*

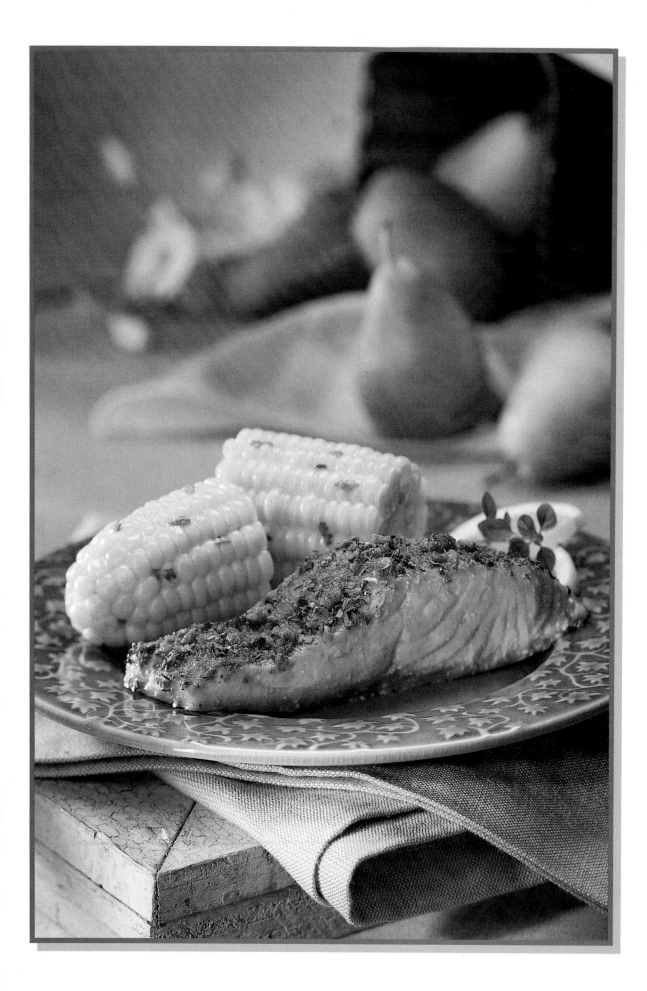

1 teaspoon canola oil
¼ cup chopped onion
1 clove garlic, minced
2½ cups fat-free reduced-sodium chicken broth
¼ cup quick-cooking barley
1 tablespoon water
1 tablespoon all-purpose flour
2 reserved ears of corn from Southwest Roasted Salmon & Corn (page 130)
6 ounces reserved salmon from Southwest Roasted Salmon & Corn (page 130)
⅓ cup reduced-fat (2%) milk
1 tablespoon minced cilantro
Black pepper
Lime wedges

# Salmon, Corn & Barley Chowder

*1.* Heat oil in medium saucepan over medium heat until hot. Add onion and garlic. Cook and stir 1 to 2 minutes or until onion is tender.

*2.* Add broth and bring to a boil. Stir in barley. Cover; reduce heat to low. Simmer 10 minutes or until barley is tender.

*3.* Stir water slowly into flour in cup until smooth.

*4.* Cut kernels from ears of corn. Break salmon into chunks.

*5.* Add corn, salmon and milk to saucepan, stirring to blend. Stir in flour mixture. Simmer gently 2 to 3 minutes or until slightly thickened. Stir in cilantro and pepper. Serve with lime wedges.

*Makes 2 (2¼-cup) servings*

Nutrients per Serving: Calories: 321, Calories from Fat: 20%, Total Fat: 7 g, Saturated Fat: 1 g, Protein: 26 g, Carbohydrate: 40 g, Cholesterol: 46 mg, Sodium: 310 mg, Dietary Fiber: 7 g

Dietary Exchanges: 3 Starch, 2 Lean Meat

## Recipe Tip

Cilantro is a fresh leafy herb that has a distinctive flavor and pungent aroma. Its flavor complements spicy foods, especially Mexican, Caribbean, Thai and Vietnamese dishes.

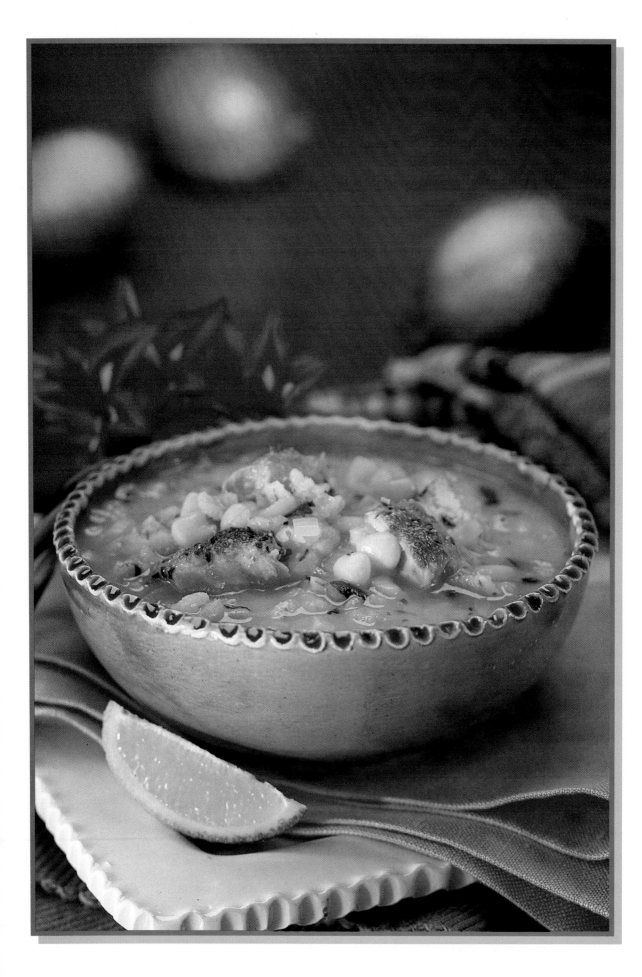

2 cups diced green
    bell peppers
2 cups thinly sliced
    carrots
2 cups thin onion
    wedges
1 pound
    mushrooms, cut
    into halves*
4 cloves garlic,
    chopped
2 tablespoons
    balsamic or red
    wine vinegar
2 teaspoons olive
    oil
¼ teaspoon salt,
    divided
¼ teaspoon black
    pepper, divided
1 tablespoon
    country-style
    Dijon mustard
1 turkey tenderloin
    (12 ounces)
1 teaspoon paprika
Nonstick cooking
    spray

*Cut large mushrooms into
quarters.

# Turkey Tenderloin with Caramelized Vegetables

1. Preheat oven to 400°F. Line 15×10-inch baking pan with heavy-duty foil.

2. Combine bell peppers, carrots, onions, mushrooms, garlic, vinegar, oil, ⅛ teaspoon salt and ⅛ teaspoon pepper in large bowl, tossing to coat vegetables evenly with seasonings. Spread vegetables onto prepared pan. Bake 15 minutes.

3. Meanwhile, spread mustard over top of turkey. Combine paprika, remaining ⅛ teaspoon salt and ⅛ teaspoon pepper in small bowl. Sprinkle over turkey. Lightly spray top of turkey with cooking spray.

4. Remove vegetables from oven. Stir vegetables and push to edges of pan. Place turkey in center of vegetables.

5. Roast 20 minutes. Stir vegetables. Roast 20 minutes more or until turkey is no longer pink in center (170°F). Let turkey stand 5 minutes. Carve half of turkey across the grain into ½-inch-thick slices. Reserve remaining turkey for Turkey Paprikash (page 135).

6. Divide sliced turkey between two plates. Place 1 cup vegetables on each plate. Reserve remaining vegetables for Turkey Paprikash (page 135).
*Makes 2 servings*

Nutrients per Serving: Calories: 232, Calories from Fat: 18%, Total Fat: 5 g, Saturated Fat: 1 g, Protein: 20 g, Carbohydrate: 30 g, Cholesterol: 34 mg, Sodium: 215 mg, Dietary Fiber: 7 g

Dietary Exchanges: 4 Vegetable, 2 Lean Meat

# Turkey Paprikash

*1.* Cook noodles according to package directions, omitting salt. Drain and keep warm.

*2.* Meanwhile, spray medium skillet with cooking spray. Heat over medium heat until hot. Add garlic and paprika. Cook and stir 30 seconds or until garlic is fragrant. Stir in water, tomato paste, salt and pepper. Simmer, uncovered, 5 minutes.

*3.* Stir in leftover turkey and vegetables. Cover; simmer 5 minutes or until heated through. Remove from heat; stir in sour cream and noodles. Top each serving with parsley.          *Makes 2 servings*

**Nutrients per Serving:** *Calories: 330, Calories from Fat: 19%, Total Fat: 7 g, Saturated Fat: 3 g, Protein: 26 g, Carbohydrate: 43 g, Cholesterol: 47 mg, Sodium: 484 mg, Dietary Fiber: 8 g*

**Dietary Exchanges:** *3 Vegetable, 2 Starch, 2 Lean Meat*

---

## Recipe Tip

For added flavor in this recipe, add tomato paste to the skillet after cooking garlic. Cook the tomato paste for 2 or 3 minutes before adding water and seasonings, then proceed with recipe as directed.

---

1 cup yolk-free extra-broad noodles
Nonstick cooking spray
2 cloves garlic, minced
2 teaspoons paprika
¾ cup water
1½ tablespoons tomato paste
⅛ teaspoon salt
⅛ teaspoon black pepper
4 ounces reserved Turkey Tenderloin (page 134), cut into ½-inch pieces
1¾ cups reserved Caramelized Vegetables (page 134)
3 tablespoons reduced-fat sour cream
2 teaspoons minced fresh parsley

# Meatless Dinners

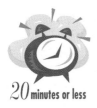

**20** minutes or less

*Need a change of pace? Try one of these tasty meatless meals.*

## Grilled Mozzarella & Roasted Red Pepper Sandwich

1 tablespoon reduced-fat olive oil vinaigrette or Italian salad dressing
2 slices (2 ounces) Italian-style sandwich bread
⅓ cup bottled roasted red peppers, rinsed, drained and patted dry
Basil leaves (optional)
2 ounces part-skim mozzarella or reduced-fat Swiss cheese slices
Nonstick olive oil cooking spray

*1.* Brush dressing on one side of one slice of bread; top with peppers, basil, if desired, cheese and second bread slice. Lightly spray both sides of sandwich with cooking spray.

*2.* Heat skillet over medium heat. Place sandwich in skillet; grill 4 to 5 minutes per side until brown and cheese is melted. *Makes 1 serving*

**Nutrients per Serving:** *Calories: 303, Calories from Fat: 29%, Total Fat: 9 g, Saturated Fat: 5 g, Protein: 16 g, Carbohydrate: 35 g, Cholesterol: 25 mg, Sodium: 727 mg, Dietary Fiber: 2 g*

**Dietary Exchanges:** *1 Vegetable, 2 Starch, 1 Lean Meat, 1½ Fat*

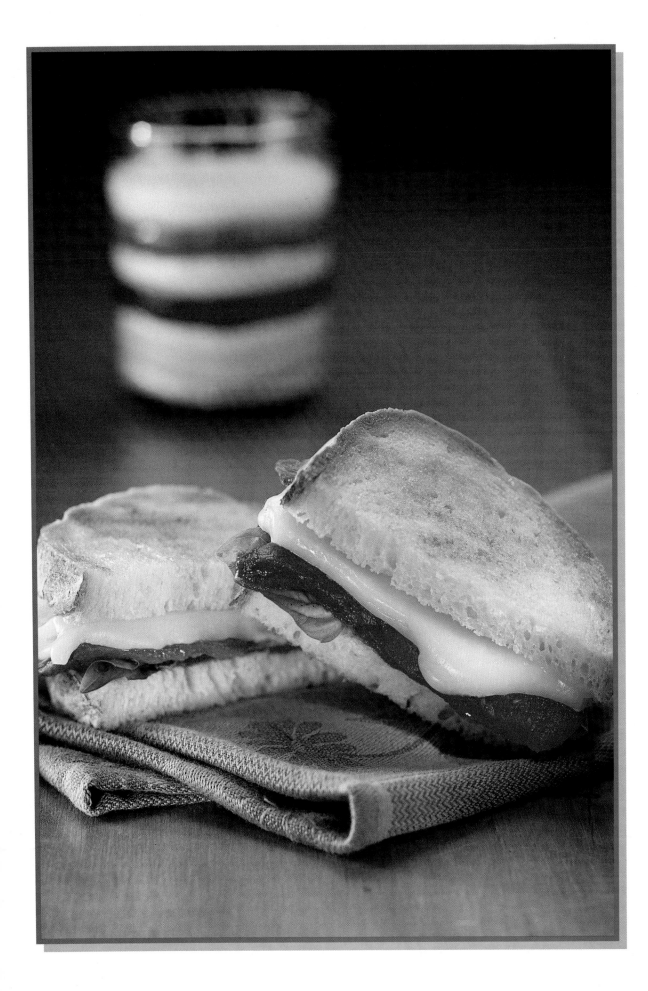

1 teaspoon olive oil
¼ cup diced green
　　bell pepper
¼ cup diced zucchini
¼ cup sliced
　　mushrooms
¼ cup diced carrot
¼ cup sliced green
　　onions
2 cloves garlic,
　　minced
1 plum tomato,
　　diced
1 tablespoon red
　　wine or water
½ teaspoon dried
　　basil leaves
¼ teaspoon salt
⅛ teaspoon black
　　pepper
2 cups cooked
　　spaghetti
　　squash
2 tablespoons
　　grated
　　Parmesan
　　cheese

# Spaghetti Squash Primavera

*1.* Heat oil in medium skillet over low heat. Add bell pepper, zucchini, mushrooms, carrot, green onions and garlic; cook 10 to 12 minutes or until crisp-tender, stirring ocassionally. Stir in tomato, wine, basil, salt and black pepper; cook 4 to 5 minutes, stirring once or twice.

*2.* Serve vegetables over spaghetti squash. Top with cheese.               *Makes 2 servings*

**Nutrients per Serving:** *Calories: 116, Calories from Fat: 32%, Total Fat: 5 g, Saturated Fat: 1 g, Protein: 5 g, Carbohydrate: 15 g, Cholesterol: 4 mg, Sodium: 396 mg, Dietary Fiber: 5 g*

**Dietary Exchanges:** *3 Vegetable, 1 Fat*

## Recipe Tip

To cook spaghetti squash, cut the squash in half lengthwise. Remove and discard seeds. Place squash, cut side down, in a 13×9-inch baking dish sprayed with nonstick cooking spray. Bake at 350°F for 45 minutes to 1 hour or until tender. Using a fork, remove spaghetti-like strands from hot squash.

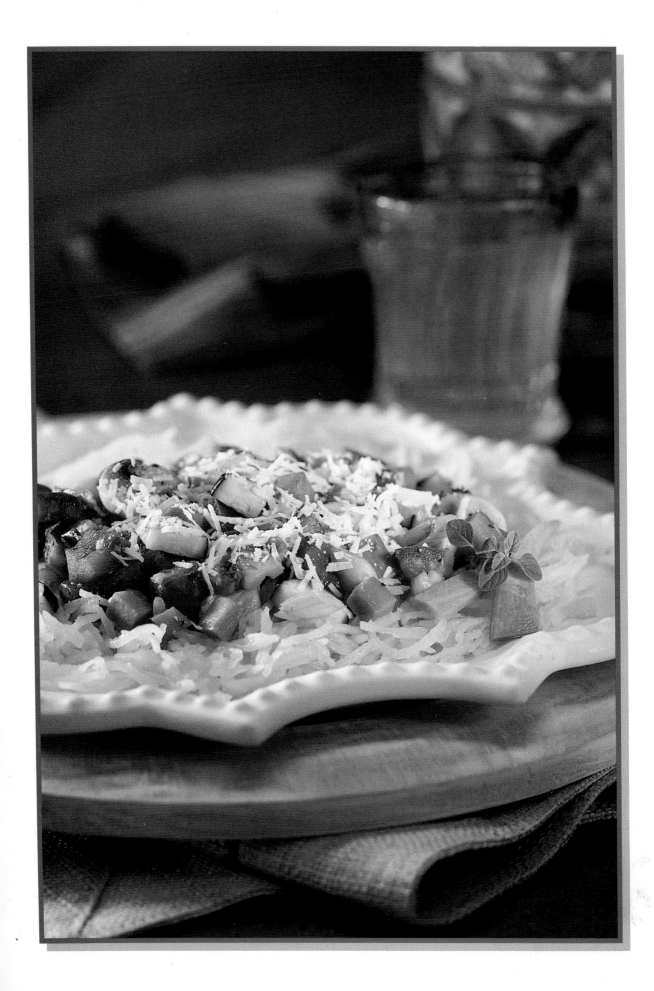

# Vegetable & Tofu Gratin

Nonstick cooking
spray
1 teaspoon olive oil
¾ cup thinly sliced
fennel bulb
¾ cup thinly sliced
onion
2 cloves garlic,
minced
¾ cup cooked brown
rice
2 tablespoons
balsamic
vinegar, divided
2 teaspoons Italian
seasoning,
divided
3 ounces firm tofu,
crumbled
¼ cup crumbled feta
cheese
6 ounces ripe plum
tomatoes, sliced
¼ inch thick
6 ounces zucchini,
sliced ¼ inch
thick
⅛ teaspoon salt
⅛ teaspoon black
pepper
¼ cup fresh bread
crumbs
2 tablespoons
grated fresh
Parmesan
cheese

*1.* Preheat oven to 400°F. Spray 1-quart shallow baking dish with nonstick cooking spray.

*2.* Spray medium skillet with cooking spray. Heat oil in skillet over medium heat until hot. Add fennel and onion. Cook about 10 minutes or until tender and lightly browned, stirring frequently. Add garlic; cook and stir 1 minute. Spread over bottom of prepared baking dish.

*3.* Combine rice, 1 tablespoon vinegar and ½ teaspoon Italian seasoning in small bowl. Spread over onion mixture.

*4.* Combine tofu, feta cheese, remaining 1 tablespoon vinegar and 1 teaspoon Italian seasoning in same small bowl; toss to combine. Spoon over rice.

*5.* Top with alternating rows of tomato and zucchini slices. Sprinkle with salt and pepper.

*6.* Combine bread crumbs, Parmesan cheese and remaining ½ teaspoon Italian seasoning in small bowl. Sprinkle over top. Spray bread crumb topping lightly with nonstick cooking spray. Bake 30 minutes or until heated through and topping is browned.

*Makes 2 servings*

**Nutrients per Serving:** *Calories: 399, Calories from Fat: 30%, Total Fat: 14 g, Saturated Fat: 5 g, Protein: 19 g, Carbohydrate: 52 g, Cholesterol: 19 mg, Sodium: 460 mg, Dietary Fiber: 7 g*

**Dietary Exchanges:** *2 Vegetable, 3 Starch, 3 Fat*

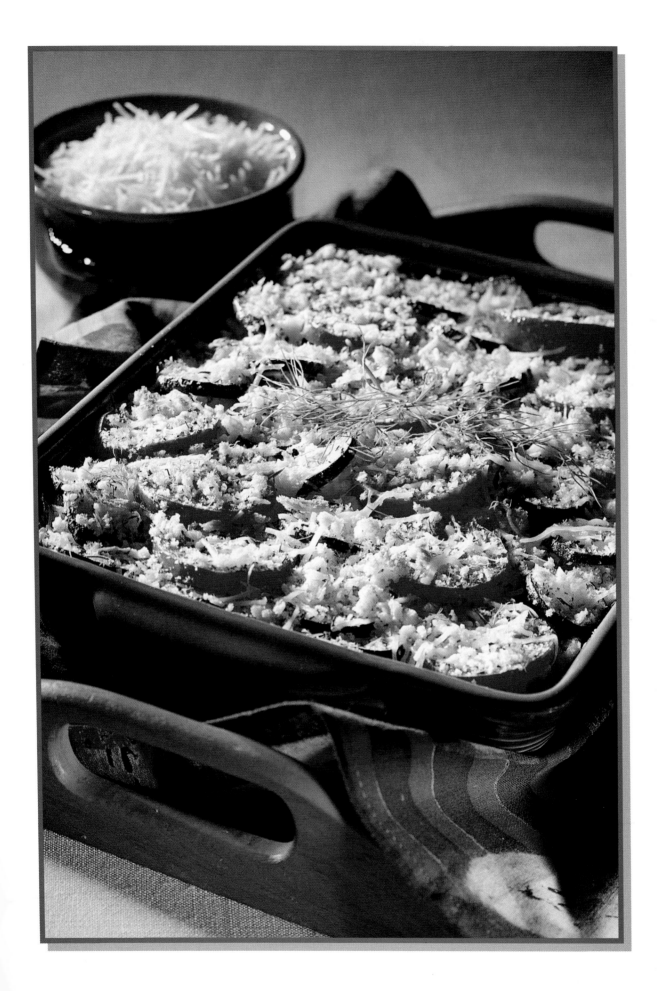

1 teaspoon olive oil
½ cup diced red bell
    pepper
¼ cup diced onion
1¼ teaspoons curry
    powder
1 clove garlic,
    minced
½ teaspoon salt
1¼ cups peeled,
    cubed eggplant
¾ cup peeled, cubed
    acorn or
    butternut
    squash
⅔ cup rinsed and
    drained canned
    chick-peas
½ cup vegetable
    broth or water
3 tablespoons white
    wine
  Hot pepper sauce
    (optional)
¼ cup lemon-
    flavored sugar-
    free yogurt
2 tablespoons
    chopped fresh
    parsley

# Curried Eggplant, Squash & Chick-Pea Stew

*1.* Heat oil in medium saucepan over medium heat. Add bell pepper and onion; cook and stir 5 minutes. Stir in curry powder, garlic and salt. Add eggplant, squash, chick-peas, broth and wine to saucepan. Cover; bring to a boil. Reduce heat and simmer 20 to 25 minutes just until squash and eggplant are tender.

*2.* Season to taste with pepper sauce, if desired. Serve with yogurt and parsley.       *Makes 2 servings*

Nutrients per Serving: *Calories: 216, Calories from Fat: 14%, Total Fat: 4 g, Saturated Fat: <1 g, Protein: 7 g, Carbohydrate: 38g, Cholesterol: 0 mg, Sodium: 47 mg, Dietary Fiber: 10 g*

Dietary Exchanges: *2½ Starch, 1 Fat*

---

## Recipe Tip

Foods that are high in fiber, such as beans, whole grains, fruit and vegetables, may help lower blood glucose levels slightly in some individuals with type 2 diabetes.

---

# French Bread Portobello Pizza

*1.* Preheat oven to 450°F. Spray small skillet with cooking spray. Heat over medium-low heat until hot. Cook and stir mushroom and garlic 5 to 7 minutes or until mushroom is slightly soft.

*2.* Stir in tomato and tomato sauce; cook 5 minutes. Spread mixture over cut sides of bread. Sprinkle with cheese. Bake 15 minutes until cheese is melted. Sprinkle with pepper flakes, if desired.

*Makes 1 serving*

**Nutrients per Serving:** *Calories: 246, Calories from Fat: 13%, Total Fat: 4 g, Saturated Fat: 1 g, Protein: 15 g, Carbohydrate: 39 g, Cholesterol: 4 mg, Sodium: 661 mg, Dietary Fiber: 4 g*

**Dietary Exchanges:** *2 Vegetable, 2 Starch, 1 Lean Meat*

Nonstick cooking spray
⅓ cup sliced portobello mushroom
1 clove garlic, minced
½ cup chopped tomato
1 tablespoon tomato sauce
1 (2-ounce) piece French bread, cut in half lengthwise
¼ cup (1 ounce) shredded reduced-fat Italian blend or part-skim mozzarella cheese
Red pepper flakes (optional)

---

## Recipe Tip

Portobello mushrooms have very large dark brown caps and thick, tough stems. Because they have a firm texture when cooked, they are sometimes substituted for beef in vegetarian dishes. Baby portobello mushrooms, which are available in some produce markets, are a good choice for this recipe.

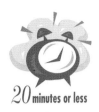

*20* minutes or less

2 tablespoons fresh lime juice
1½ teaspoons canola oil
½ teaspoon ground cumin
½ teaspoon water
⅛ teaspoon salt
¾ cup canned red beans, rinsed and drained
½ cup frozen corn with bell pepper and onion, thawed
¼ cup chopped tomato
2 tablespoons chopped green onion, divided
2 large romaine lettuce leaves

# Red Bean & Corn Salad with Lime-Cumin Dressing

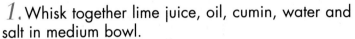

*1.* Whisk together lime juice, oil, cumin, water and salt in medium bowl.

*2.* Add beans, corn, tomato and 1 tablespoon green onion; toss to coat. Serve on lettuce leaves. Top with remaining green onion.          *Makes 1 serving*

**Nutrients per Serving:** *Calories: 198, Calories from Fat: 18%, Total Fat: 4 g, Saturated Fat: <1 g, Protein: 8 g, Carbohydrate: 33 g, Cholesterol: 0 mg, Sodium: 908 mg, Dietary Fiber: 9 g*

**Dietary Exchanges:** *2 Starch, 1 Lean Meat*

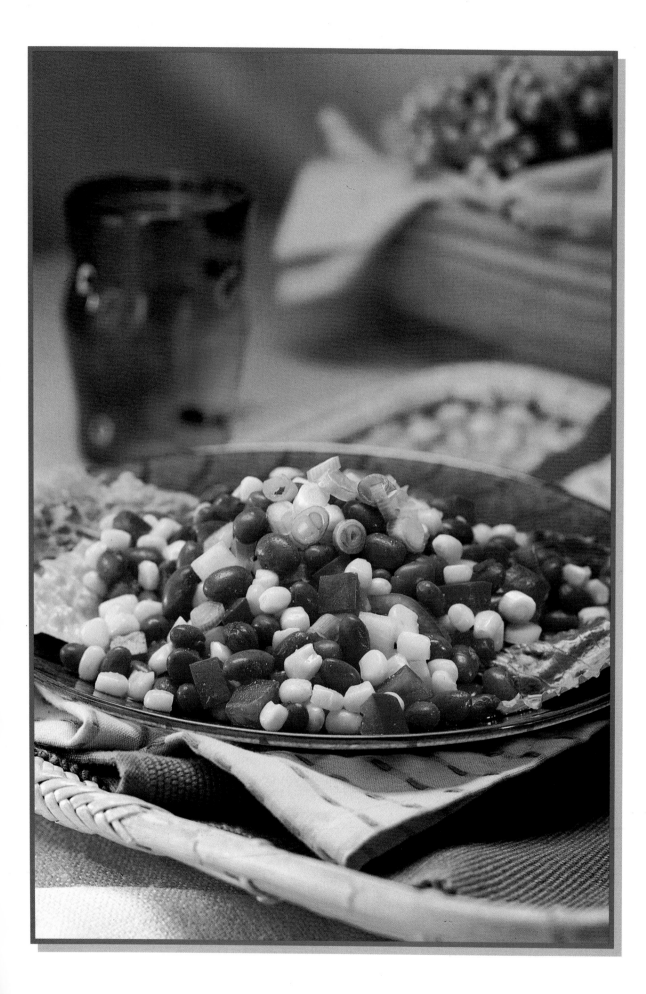

# Cheesy Baked Barley

2 cups water
½ cup medium
   pearled barley
½ teaspoon salt,
   divided
   Nonstick cooking
   spray
½ cup diced onion
½ cup diced zucchini
½ cup diced red bell
   pepper
1½ teaspoons all-
   purpose flour
   Seasoned pepper
¾ cup fat-free (skim)
   milk
1 cup (4 ounces)
   shredded
   reduced-fat
   Italian blend
   cheese, divided
1 tablespoon Dijon
   mustard

*1.* Bring water to a boil in 1-quart saucepan. Add barley and ¼ teaspoon salt. Cover and reduce heat. Simmer 45 minutes or until tender and most water is evaporated. Let stand, covered, 5 minutes.

*2.* Preheat oven to 375°F. Spray medium skillet with cooking spray. Cook onion, zucchini and bell pepper over medium-low heat about 10 minutes or until soft. Stir in flour, remaining ¼ teaspoon salt and seasoned pepper; cook 1 to 2 minutes. Add milk, stirring constantly; cook and stir until slightly thickened. Remove from heat and add barley, ¾ cup cheese and mustard; stir until cheese is melted.

*3.* Spread in even layer in casserole. Sprinkle with remaining ¼ cup cheese. Bake 20 minutes or until hot. Preheat broiler. Broil casserole 1 to 2 minutes until cheese is lightly browned.     *Makes 2 servings*

**Nutrients per Serving:** *Calories: 362, Calories from Fat: 23%, Total Fat: 9 g, Saturated Fat: 4 g, Protein: 20 g, Carbohydrate: 50 g, Cholesterol: 32 mg, Sodium: 1159 mg, Dietary Fiber: 6 g*

**Dietary Exchanges:** *2 Vegetable, 2½ Starch, 2 Lean Meat, ½ Fat*

## Recipe Tip

Barley is an excellent substitute for rice. When cooked, it has a slightly chewy texture and mild nutty flavor. Not only does it have four times the fiber of white rice, but barley also contains 20 percent less carbohydrate than white rice.

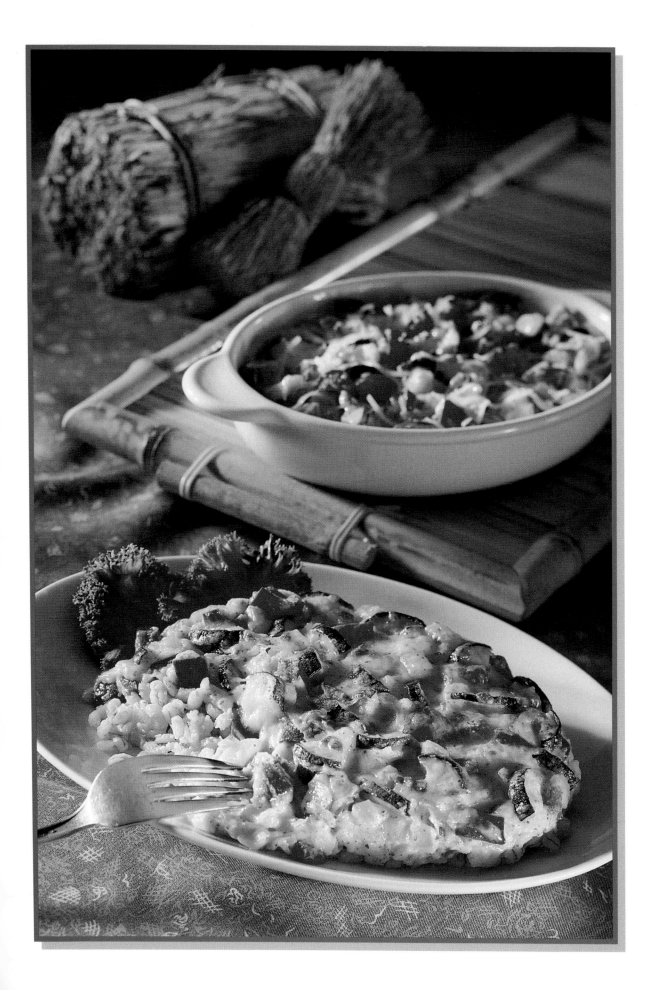

# Orange Ginger Tofu & Noodles

⅔ cup orange juice
3 tablespoons reduced-sodium soy sauce
½ to 1 teaspoon minced ginger
1 clove garlic, minced
¼ teaspoon red pepper flakes
5 ounces extra-firm tofu, well drained and cut into ½-inch cubes
1½ teaspoons cornstarch
1 teaspoon canola or peanut oil
2 cups fresh cut-up vegetables, such as broccoli, carrot, onion and snow peas
1½ cups hot cooked vermicelli pasta

*1.* Combine orange juice, soy sauce, ginger, garlic and red pepper in resealable plastic food storage bag; add tofu. Marinate 20 to 30 minutes. Drain tofu, reserving marinade. Stir marinade into cornstarch until smooth.

*2.* Heat oil in large nonstick skillet or wok over medium-high heat. Add vegetables; stir-fry 2 to 3 minutes or until vegetables are crisp-tender. Add tofu; stir-fry 1 minute. Stir reserved marinade mixture; add to skillet. Bring to a boil; boil 1 minute. Serve over vermicelli.

*Makes 2 servings*

**Nutrients per Serving:** *Calories: 305, Calories from Fat: 20%, Total Fat: 7 g, Saturated Fat: 1 g, Protein: 19 g, Carbohydrate: 42 g, Cholesterol: 0 mg, Sodium: 824 mg, Dietary Fiber: 6 g*

**Dietary Exchanges:** *2 Vegetable, 2 Starch, 1 Lean Meat, 1 Fat*

---

## Recipe Tip

To drain tofu, place it in a colander and let it stand for 5 minutes, then place it on several layers of paper towels. If extra-firm tofu is not available, use firm tofu; drain as directed above, cover with paper towels and place a small heavy plate on top. Let stand for 5 or 10 minutes, then cut into cubes.

---

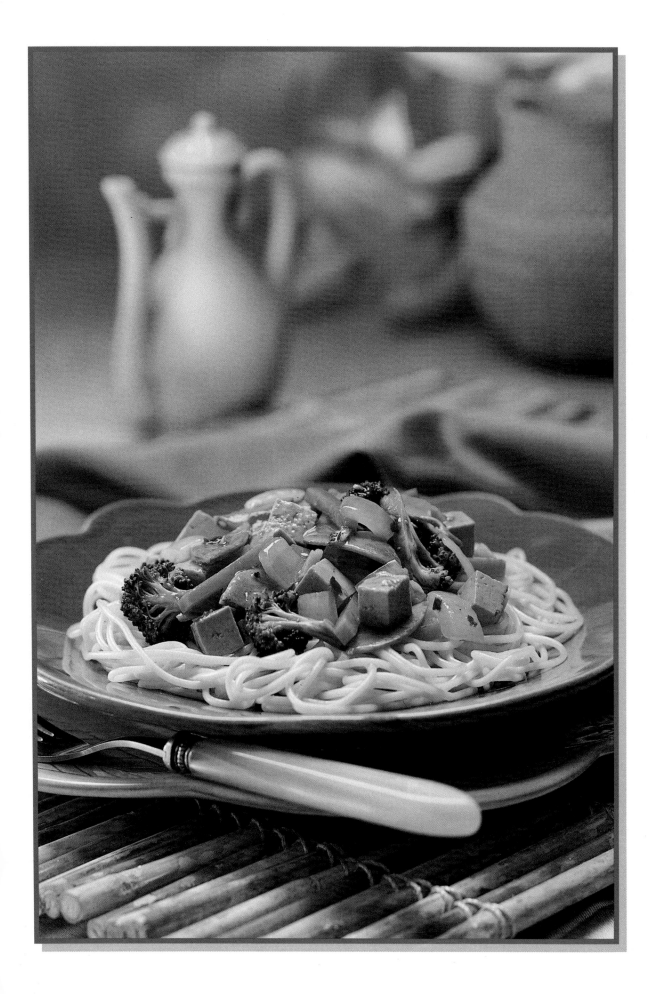

# Delicious Desserts

*You'll love these easy-to-prepare low-sugar desserts.*

## Baked Pear Dessert

2 tablespoons dried cranberries or raisins
1 tablespoon toasted sliced almonds
⅛ teaspoon cinnamon
⅓ cup unsweetened apple cider or apple juice, divided
1 medium (6 ounces) unpeeled pear, cut in half lengthwise and cored
½ cup vanilla sugar-free low-fat ice cream

*1.* Preheat oven to 350°F. Combine cranberries, almonds, cinnamon and 1 teaspoon cider in bowl.

*2.* Place pear halves, cut side up, in small baking dish. Mound almond mixture on top of pear halves. Pour remaining cider into dish. Cover with foil.

*3.* Bake pear halves 35 to 40 minutes or until pears are soft, spooning cider in dish over pears once or twice during baking. Serve warm and top with ice cream. *Makes 2 servings*

**Nutrients per Serving:** *Calories: 87, Calories from Fat: 19%, Total Fat: 2 g, Saturated Fat: <1 g, Protein: 1 g, Carbohydrate: 16 g, Cholesterol: 3 mg, Sodium: 13 mg, Dietary Fiber: 1 g*

**Dietary Exchanges:** *1 Fruit, ½ Fat*

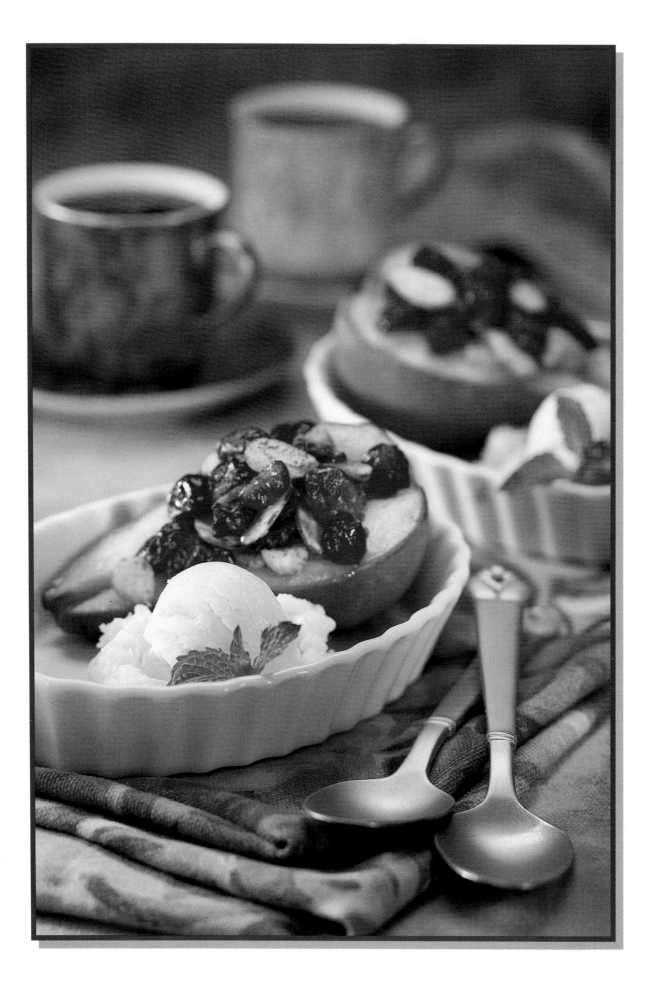

1½ tablespoons
   gingersnap
   crumbs
   (2 snaps)
¼ teaspoon ground
   ginger
2 ounces reduced-
   fat cream
   cheese,
   softened
1 container
   (6 ounces)
   peach sugar-
   free, nonfat
   yogurt
¼ teaspoon vanilla
⅓ cup chopped fresh
   peach or
   drained canned
   peaches in juice

# *Peaches & Cream Gingersnap Cups*

*1.* Combine gingersnap crumbs and ginger in small bowl; set aside.

*2.* Beat cream cheese in small bowl at medium speed of electric mixer until smooth. Add yogurt and vanilla. Beat at low speed until smooth and well blended. Stir in chopped peach.

*3.* Divide peach mixture between two 6-ounce custard cups. Cover and refrigerate 1 hour. Top each serving with half of gingersnap crumb mixture just before serving.           *Makes 2 servings*

**Note:** Instead of crushing the gingersnaps, serve them whole with the peaches & cream cups.

Nutrients per Serving: *Calories: 148, Calories from Fat: 34%, Total Fat: 5 g, Saturated Fat: 3 g, Protein: 6 g, Carbohydrate: 18 g, Cholesterol: 16 mg, Sodium: 204 mg, Dietary Fiber: 1 g*

Dietary Exchanges: *1 Starch, ½ Milk, 1 Fat*

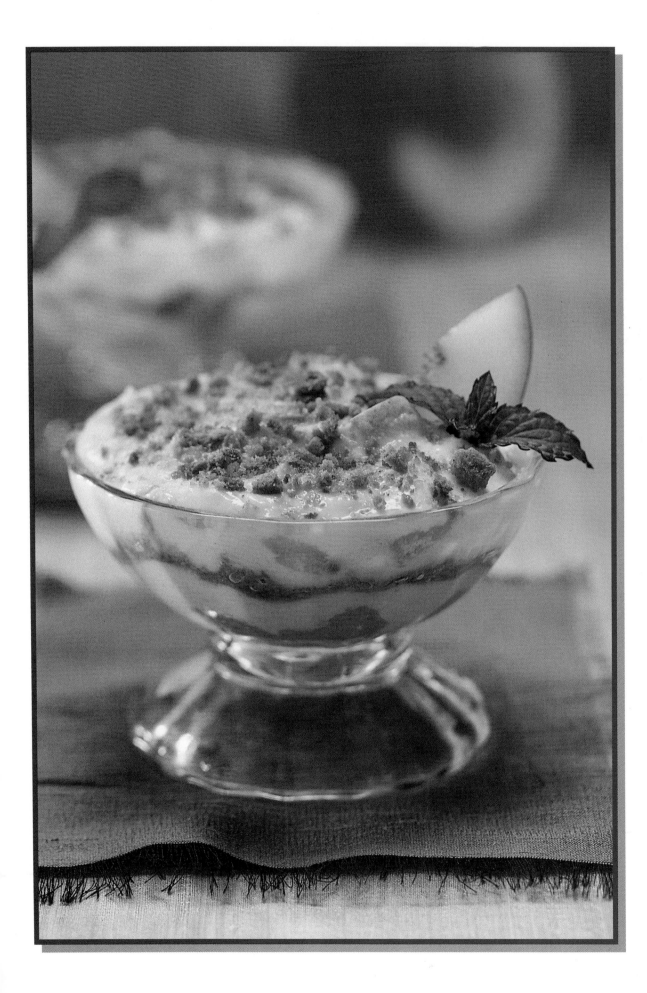

# Easy Citrus Berry Shortcake

1 individual sponge
cake
1 tablespoon
orange juice
¼ cup lemon chiffon
sugar-free,
nonfat yogurt
¼ cup thawed
frozen fat-free
nondairy
whipped
topping
⅔ cup sliced
strawberries or
raspberries
Mint leaves
(optional)

*1.* Place individual sponge cake on serving plate. Drizzle with orange juice.

*2.* Fold together yogurt and whipped topping. Spoon half of mixture onto cake. Top with berries and remaining yogurt mixture. Garnish with mint leaves.                    *Makes 1 serving*

**Nutrients per Serving:** *Calories: 173, Calories from Fat: 7%, Total Fat: 1 g, Saturated Fat: <1 g, Protein: 4 g, Carbohydrate: 37 g, Cholesterol: 39 mg, Sodium: 116 mg, Dietary Fiber: 3 g*

**Dietary Exchanges:** *1 Fruit, 1½ Starch*

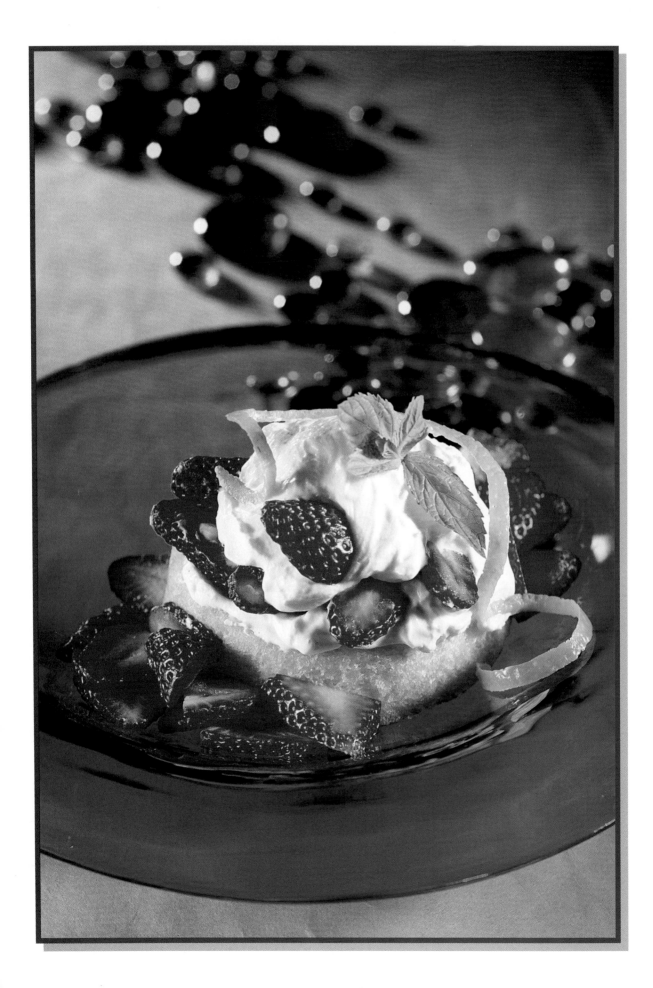

# Peach Custard

½ cup peeled fresh
   peach or
   nectarine, cut
   into chunks
1 can (5 ounces)
   evaporated
   skimmed milk*
¼ cup cholesterol-
   free egg
   substitute
1 packet sugar
   substitute or
   equivalent of
   2 teaspoons
   sugar
½ teaspoon vanilla
   Cinnamon

*If a 5-ounce can is not
available, use ½ cup plus
2 tablespoons evaporated
skimmed milk.

*1.* Preheat oven to 325°F. Divide peach chunks between two 6-ounce ovenproof custard cups. Whisk together milk, egg substitute, sugar substitute and vanilla. Pour mixture over peach chunks in custard cups.

*2.* Place custard cups in shallow 1-quart casserole. Carefully pour hot water into casserole to depth of 1-inch. Bake custards 50 minutes or until knife inserted in center comes out clean. Remove custard cups from water bath. Serve warm or at room temperature; sprinkle with cinnamon.

*Makes 2 servings*

**Note:** Drained canned peach slices in juice may be substituted for fresh fruit.

Nutrients per Serving: *Calories: 52, Calories from Fat: 2%, Total Fat: <1 g, Saturated Fat: <1 g, Protein: 5 g, Carbohydrate: 7g, Cholesterol: <1 mg, Sodium: 71 mg, Dietary Fiber: 1 g*

Dietary Exchanges: *1 Fruit*

---

## Recipe Tip

Since about half the water is removed from fat-free milk to produce evaporated skimmed milk, it has more flavor than fresh milk. If you don't like the slightly caramelized flavor of canned milk in a recipe, substitute fresh fat-free milk.

# Cinnamon Compote

½ cup unsweetened
  pineapple juice
⅛ teaspoon ground
  cinnamon
1½ cups cubed
  cantaloupe
½ cup blueberries

*1.* In small saucepan combine juice and cinnamon. Cook and stir over low heat 4 to 5 minutes or until slightly syrupy. Cool slightly.

*2.* Combine cantaloupe and blueberries. Pour juice mixture over fruit; toss. Refrigerate until cold.

*Makes 2 servings*

**Nutrients per Serving:** *Calories: 98, Calories from Fat: 4%, Total Fat: 1 g, Saturated Fat: <1 g, Protein: 2 g, Carbohydrate: 24 g, Cholesterol: 0 mg, Sodium: 14 mg, Dietary Fiber: 2 g*

**Dietary Exchanges:** *1½ Fruit*

---

## Recipe Tip

This recipe is an easy way to dress up summer fruit, such as vitamin A-rich cantaloupe.

---

½ cup fresh
blueberries
2 tablespoons all-
purpose flour
1½ tablespoons
granulated
sugar
⅛ teaspoon salt
¼ teaspoon ground
cardamom
¼ cup cholesterol-
free egg
substitute
1 teaspoon grated
lemon peel
½ teaspoon vanilla
¾ cup reduced-fat
(2%) milk
1 teaspoon
powdered sugar

# Blueberry Custard Supreme

*1.* Preheat oven to 350°F. Spray 1-quart soufflé or casserole dish with nonstick cooking spray. Distribute blueberries over bottom of prepared dish.

*2.* Whisk flour, granulated sugar, salt and cardamom in small bowl. Add egg substitute, lemon peel and vanilla; whisk until smooth and well blended. Whisk in milk. Pour over blueberries.

*3.* Bake 30 minutes or until puffed, lightly browned and center is set. Cool on wire rack. Serve warm or at room temperature. Sprinkle with powdered sugar just before serving.  *Makes 2 servings*

**Blackberry Custard Supreme:** Substitute fresh blackberries for blueberries; proceed as directed.

**Nutrients per Serving:** *Calories: 155, Calories from Fat: 11%, Total Fat: 2 g, Saturated Fat: 1 g, Protein: 7 g, Carbohydrate: 27g, Cholesterol: 7 mg, Sodium: 249 mg, Dietary Fiber: 1 g*

**Dietary Exchanges:** *½ Fruit, 1 Starch, ½ Milk*

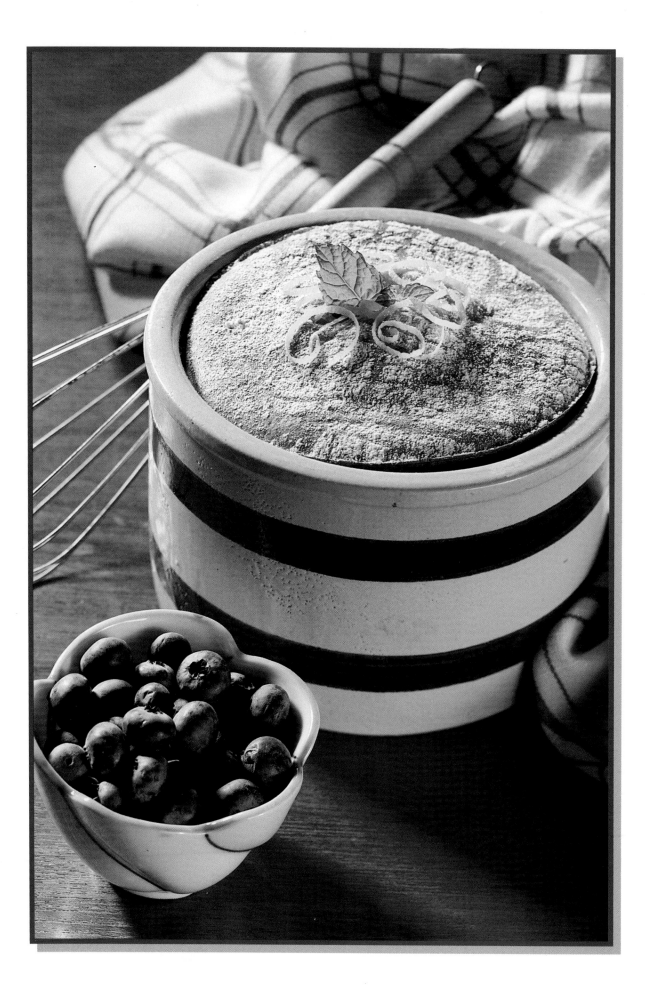

½ cup day-old
   French bread
   cubes
1 tablespoon dried
   cranberries or
   tart cherries
⅓ cup fat-free (skim)
   milk
1 tablespoon
   refrigerated
   cholesterol-free
   egg substitute
1 tablespoon brown
   sugar
¼ teaspoon vanilla
⅛ teaspoon ground
   cinnamon

# Cranberry Bread Pudding

*1.* Preheat oven to 350°F. Toss together bread cubes and cranberries. Place in 6-ounce custard cup.

*2.* Stir together milk, egg substitute, brown sugar, vanilla and cinnamon. Pour over bread mixture. Bake 22 to 25 minutes or until knife inserted in center comes out clean. Cool slightly.          *Makes 1 serving*

**Nutrients per Serving:** *Calories: 163, Calories from Fat: 5%, Total Fat: 1 g, Saturated Fat: <1 g, Protein: 6 g, Carbohydrate: 33 g, Cholesterol: 1 mg, Sodium: 151 mg, Dietary Fiber: 1 g*

**Dietary Exchanges:** *1½ Starch, ½ Milk*

---

## Recipe Tip

Since cranberries are very tart, a little granulated sugar is added to them during processing. Dried tart cherries are not sweetened and are a good substitute for dried cranberries. However, dried tart cherries are not readily available. If they are not available in your supermarket, look for them in gourmet food stores or catalogues.

---

# *Diabetic* DESSERTS

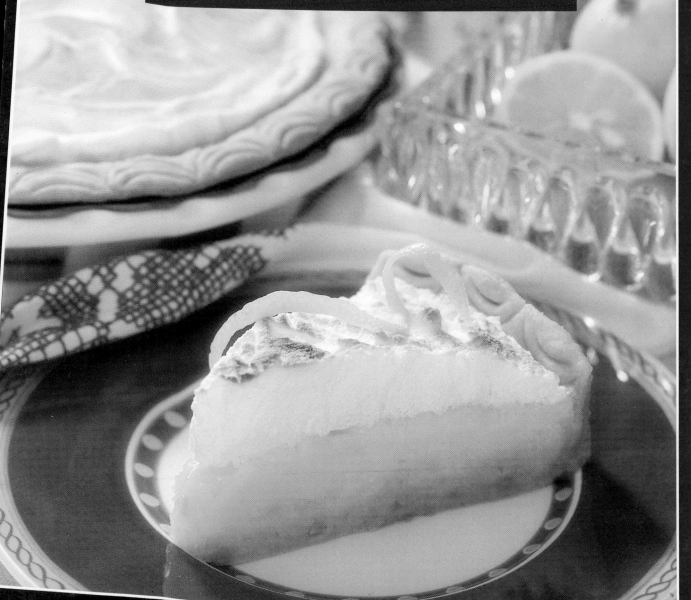

# Diabetic Desserts

# Everyday Delights

## Chocolate Fudge Cheesecake Parfaits

1½ cups nonfat cottage cheese
    4 packets sugar substitute *or* equivalent of 8 teaspoons sugar
    2 teaspoons packed brown sugar
1½ teaspoons vanilla
    2 tablespoons semisweet mini chocolate chips, divided
    2 cups fat-free chocolate ice cream or fat-free frozen yogurt
    3 tablespoons graham cracker crumbs

**1.** Combine cottage cheese, sugar substitute, brown sugar and vanilla in food processor or blender; process until smooth. Stir in 1 tablespoon mini chips with wooden spoon.

**2.** Spoon about ¼ cup ice cream into each stemmed glass. Top with heaping tablespoon cheese mixture; sprinkle with 2 teaspoons graham cracker crumbs. Repeat layers. Freeze parfaits 15 to 30 minutes to firm slightly.

**3.** Garnish each parfait with remaining 1 tablespoon mini chips and remaining cracker crumbs.

*Makes 4 servings*

### Nutrients per Serving

| | | | | | |
|---|---|---|---|---|---|
| Calories | 199 | Saturated Fat | 1 g | Cholesterol | 0 mg |
| Calories from Fat | 11 % | Protein | 17 g | Sodium | 419 mg |
| Total Fat | 2 g | Carbohydrate | 28 g | Dietary Fiber | 1 g |

DIETARY EXCHANGES: 1½ Starch, 1½ Lean Meat

*Chocolate Fudge Cheesecake Parfaits*

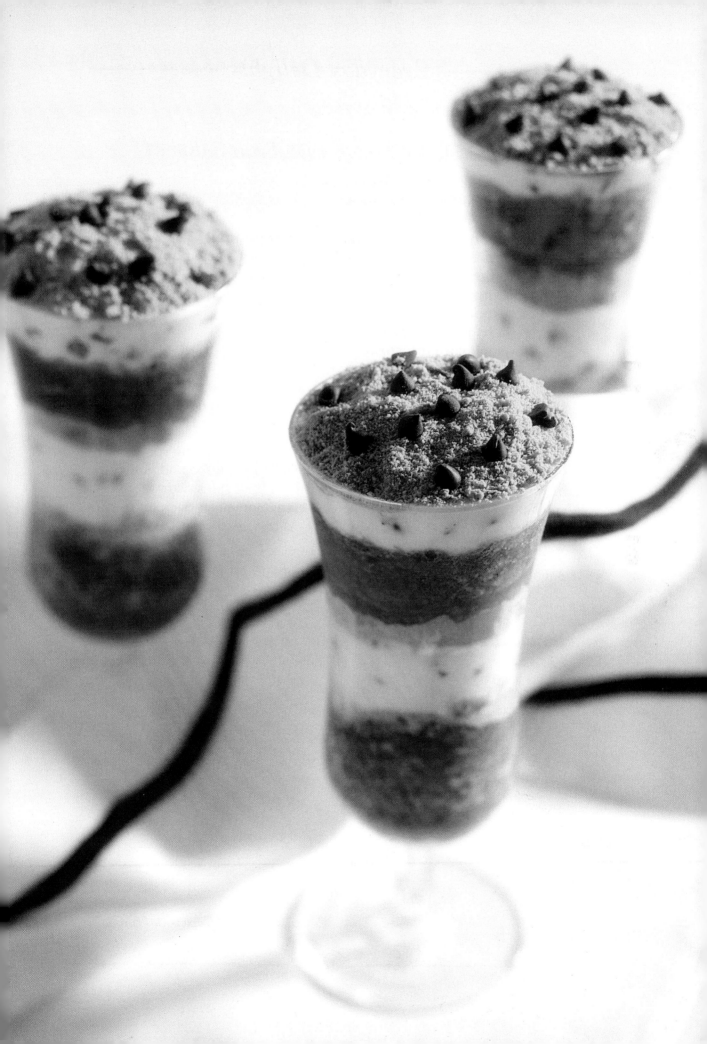

## Cinnamon Dessert Tacos with Fruit Salsa

**1 cup sliced fresh strawberries**
**1 cup cubed fresh pineapple**
**1 cup cubed peeled kiwi**
**½ teaspoon minced jalapeño pepper (optional)**
**2 packets sugar substitute *or* equivalent of 4 teaspoons sugar (optional)**
**3 tablespoons sugar**
**1 tablespoon ground cinnamon**
**6 (8-inch) flour tortillas**
**Nonstick cooking spray**

**1.** Stir together strawberries, pineapple, kiwi, jalapeño pepper and sugar substitute in large bowl; set aside. Combine sugar and cinnamon in small bowl; set aside.

**2.** Spray tortilla lightly on both sides with nonstick cooking spray. Heat over medium heat in nonstick skillet until slightly puffed and golden brown. Remove from heat; immediately dust both sides with cinnamon-sugar mixture. Shake excess cinnamon-sugar back into small bowl. Repeat cooking and dusting process until all tortillas are warmed.

**3.** Fold tortillas in half and fill with fruit mixture. Serve immediately.

*Makes 6 servings*

### Nutrients per Serving

| | | | | | |
|---|---|---|---|---|---|
| Calories | 183 | Saturated Fat | <1 g | Cholesterol | 0 mg |
| Calories from Fat | 14% | Protein | 4 g | Sodium | 169 mg |
| Total Fat | 3 g | Carbohydrate | 36 g | Dietary Fiber | 4 g |

DIETARY EXCHANGES: 1½ Starch, 1 Fruit, ½ Fat

*Cinnamon Dessert Taco with Fruit Salsa*

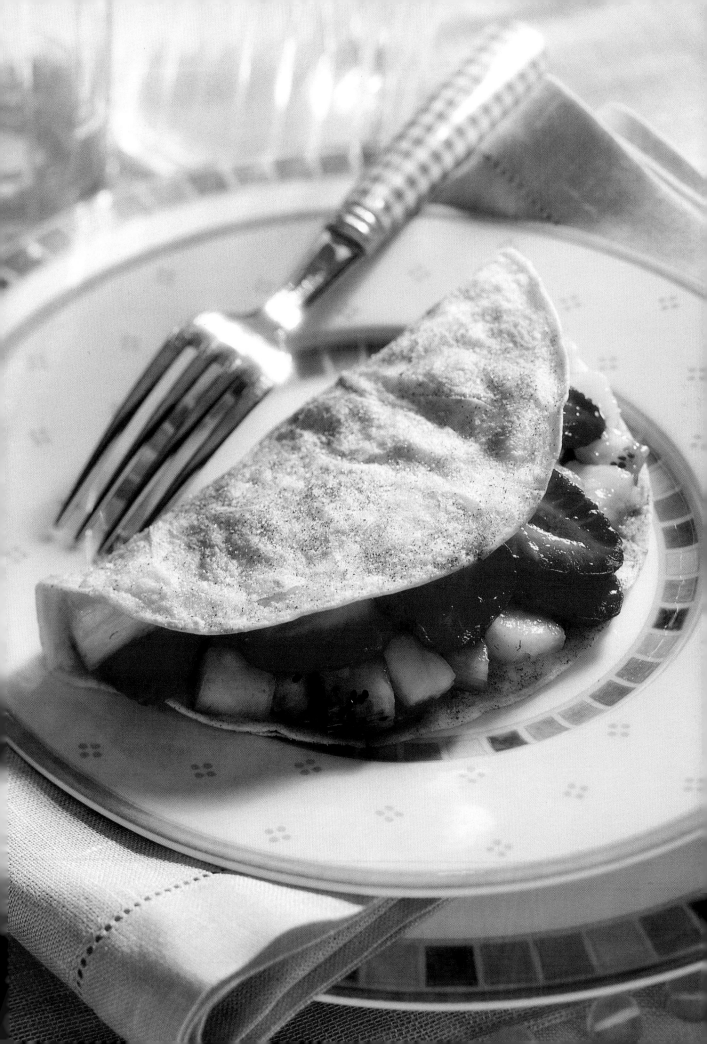

## New Age Candy Apple

**1 Granny Smith apple, peeled**
**¼ teaspoon sugar-free cherry-flavored gelatin**
**2 tablespoons diet cherry cola**
**2 tablespoons thawed frozen reduced-fat nondairy whipped topping**

**1.** Slice apple crosswise into ¼-inch-thick rings; remove seeds. Place stack of apple rings in small microwavable bowl; sprinkle with gelatin. Pour cola over rings.

**2.** Cover loosely with waxed paper. Microwave at HIGH 2 minutes or until liquid is boiling. Allow to stand, covered, 5 minutes. Arrange rings on dessert plate. Serve warm with whipped topping.

*Makes 1 serving*

**Note:** This recipe can be doubled or tripled easily. To cook 2 apples at a time, increase cooking time to 3½ minutes. To cook 3 apples at a time, increase cooking time to 5 minutes.

### Nutrients per Serving

| | | | | | |
|---|---|---|---|---|---|
| Calories | 102 | Saturated Fat | 1 g | Cholesterol | 0 mg |
| Calories from Fat | 17 % | Protein | <1 g | Sodium | 1 mg |
| Total Fat | 2 g | Carbohydrate | 23 g | Dietary Fiber | 4 g |

DIETARY EXCHANGES: 1½ Fruit

*This recipe works great with any crisp apple. A Jonathan apple will give a tart flavor, a Cortland apple will give a sweet-tart flavor and a Red Delicious apple will give a sweet flavor. Choose your favorite apple and enjoy!*

*New Age Candy Apple*

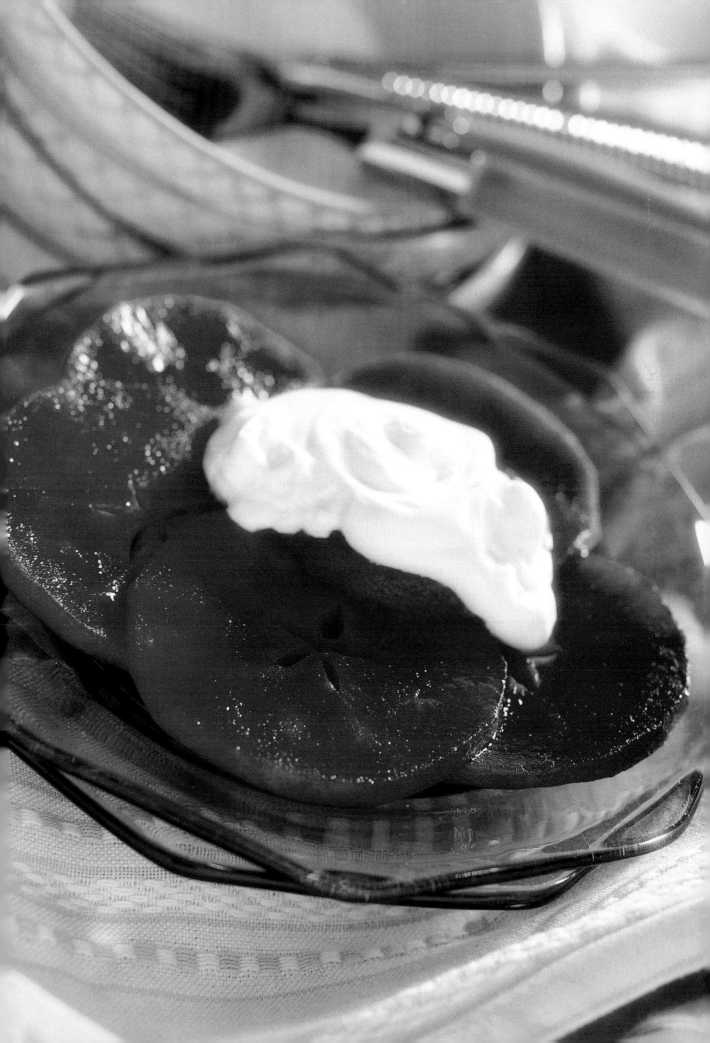

## Rocky Road Pudding

¼ cup sugar
5 tablespoons unsweetened cocoa powder
3 tablespoons cornstarch
⅛ teaspoon salt
2½ cups low-fat (1%) milk
2 egg yolks, beaten
2 teaspoons vanilla
6 packets sugar substitute *or* equivalent of ¼ cup sugar
1 cup miniature marshmallows
¼ cup chopped walnuts, toasted

**1.** Combine sugar, cocoa, cornstarch and salt in small saucepan; mix well. Stir in milk; cook over medium-high heat, stirring constantly, about 10 minutes or until mixture thickens and begins to boil.

**2.** Pour about ½ cup pudding mixture over beaten egg yolks in small bowl; beat well. Pour mixture back into saucepan. Cook over medium heat an additional 10 minutes. Remove from heat; stir in vanilla.

**3.** Place plastic wrap on surface of pudding. Refrigerate about 20 minutes or until slightly cooled. Remove plastic wrap; stir in sugar substitute. Spoon pudding into 6 dessert dishes; top with marshmallows and nuts. Serve warm or cold.          *Makes 6 servings*

### Nutrients per Serving

| | | | | | |
|---|---|---|---|---|---|
| Calories | 190 | Saturated Fat | 1 g | Cholesterol | 75 mg |
| Calories from Fat | 27 % | Protein | 7 g | Sodium | 121 mg |
| Total Fat | 6 g | Carbohydrate | 28 g | Dietary Fiber | <1 g |

DIETARY EXCHANGES: 1 Starch, ½ Milk, 1 Fat

## Cranberry-Orange Bread Pudding

**2 cups cubed cinnamon bread**
**¼ cup dried cranberries**
**2 cups low-fat (1%) milk**
**1 package (4 serving size) sugar-free vanilla pudding and pie filling mix\***
**½ cup cholesterol-free egg substitute**
**1 teaspoon vanilla**
**1 teaspoon grated orange peel**
**½ teaspoon ground cinnamon**
   **Low-fat no-sugar-added vanilla ice cream (optional)**

*\*Do not use instant pudding and pie filling.*

**1.** Preheat oven to 325°F. Spray 9 custard cups with nonstick cooking spray.

**2.** Place bread cubes in custard cups. Bake 10 minutes; add cranberries.

**3.** Combine remaining ingredients except ice cream in medium bowl. Carefully pour over mixture in custard cups. Let stand 5 to 10 minutes.

**4.** Place cups on baking sheet; bake 25 to 30 minutes or until center is almost set. Let stand 10 minutes. Serve with ice cream, if desired.

*Makes 9 servings*

### Nutrients per Serving

| | | | | | |
|---|---|---|---|---|---|
| Calories | 67 | Saturated Fat | <1 g | Cholesterol | 2 mg |
| Calories from Fat | 13% | Protein | 4 g | Sodium | 190 mg |
| Total Fat | 1 g | Carbohydrate | 11 g | Dietary Fiber | <1 g |

DIETARY EXCHANGES: 1 Starch

## Orange Smoothies

**1 cup fat-free vanilla ice cream or fat-free vanilla frozen yogurt**
**¾ cup low-fat (1%) milk**
**¼ cup frozen orange juice concentrate**

**1.** Combine ice cream, milk and orange juice concentrate in food processor or blender; process until smooth.

**2.** Pour mixture into 2 glasses; garnish as desired. Serve immediately.

*Makes 2 servings*

### Nutrients per Serving

| | | | | | | | |
|---|---|---|---|---|---|---|---|
| Calories | 185 | Saturated Fat | <1 g | Cholesterol | 4 mg |
| Calories from Fat | 5 % | Protein | 8 g | Sodium | 117 mg |
| Total Fat | 1 g | Carbohydrate | 38 g | Dietary Fiber | <1 g |

DIETARY EXCHANGES: 1½ Starch, 1 Fruit

## Raspberry Smoothies

**1 cup plain nonfat yogurt with aspartame sweetener**
**1 cup crushed ice**
**1½ cups fresh or frozen raspberries**
**1 tablespoon honey**
**2 packets sugar substitute *or* equivalent of 4 teaspoons sugar**

**1.** Place all ingredients in food processor or blender; process until smooth. Scrape down sides as needed. Serve immediately.

*Makes 2 servings*

### Nutrients per Serving

| | | | | | | | |
|---|---|---|---|---|---|---|---|
| Calories | 143 | Saturated Fat | <1 g | Cholesterol | 2 mg |
| Calories from Fat | 4 % | Protein | 8 g | Sodium | 88 mg |
| Total Fat | <1 g | Carbohydrate | 28 g | Dietary Fiber | 6 g |

DIETARY EXCHANGES: ½ Milk, 1½ Fruit

*Orange Smoothies*

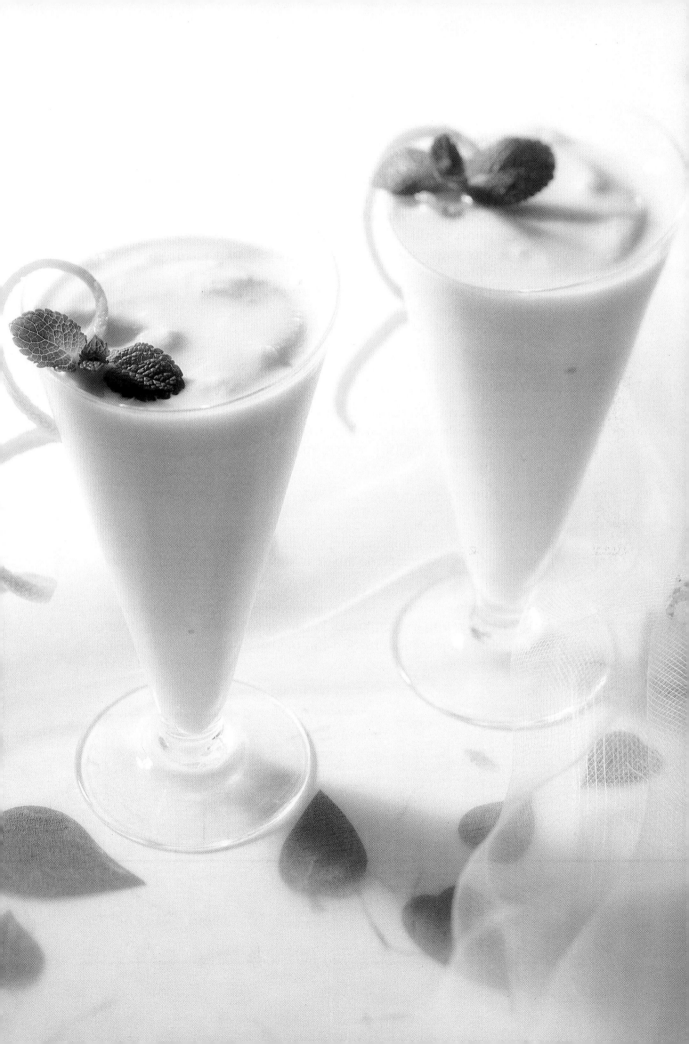

## Sugar Cookie Fruit Tart

**1 package (about 18 ounces) refrigerated sugar cookie dough**
**1 package (8 ounces) fat-free cream cheese, softened**
**¼ cup orange marmalade**
**1 teaspoon vanilla**
**2 packets sugar substitute *or* equivalent of 4 teaspoons sugar, divided**
**1 can (11 ounces) mandarin oranges, drained**
**16 strawberries, halved**
**1 kiwi, peeled, sliced and halved**

**1.** Preheat oven 350°F. Coat 12-inch pizza pan with nonstick cooking spray; set aside.

**2.** Slice dough into 16 slices. Arrange cookie slices ½ inch apart on prepared pan. Press cookie dough to cover bottom and sides of pizza pan evenly. Spray fingertips with nonstick cooking spray to prevent sticking if needed.

**3.** Bake 20 to 22 minutes or until golden brown. Cool completely in pan on wire rack.

**4.** Beat cream cheese, marmalade, vanilla and 1 packet sugar substitute in medium bowl with electric mixer at high speed until well blended; refrigerate.

**5.** To assemble, spread cream cheese mixture on top of cooled cookie crust. Mix fruit with remaining packet sugar substitute. Arrange fruit on top of cream cheese mixture. Serve immediately or cover with plastic wrap and refrigerate.                    *Makes 12 servings*

### Nutrients per Serving

| Calories | 265 | Saturated Fat | 3 g | Cholesterol | 15 mg |
|---|---|---|---|---|---|
| Calories from Fat | 34 % | Protein | 5 g | Sodium | 304 mg |
| Total Fat | 10 g | Carbohydrate | 39 g | Dietary Fiber | 2 g |

DIETARY EXCHANGES: 1½ Starch, 1 Fruit, 2 Fat

*Sugar Cookie Fruit Tart*

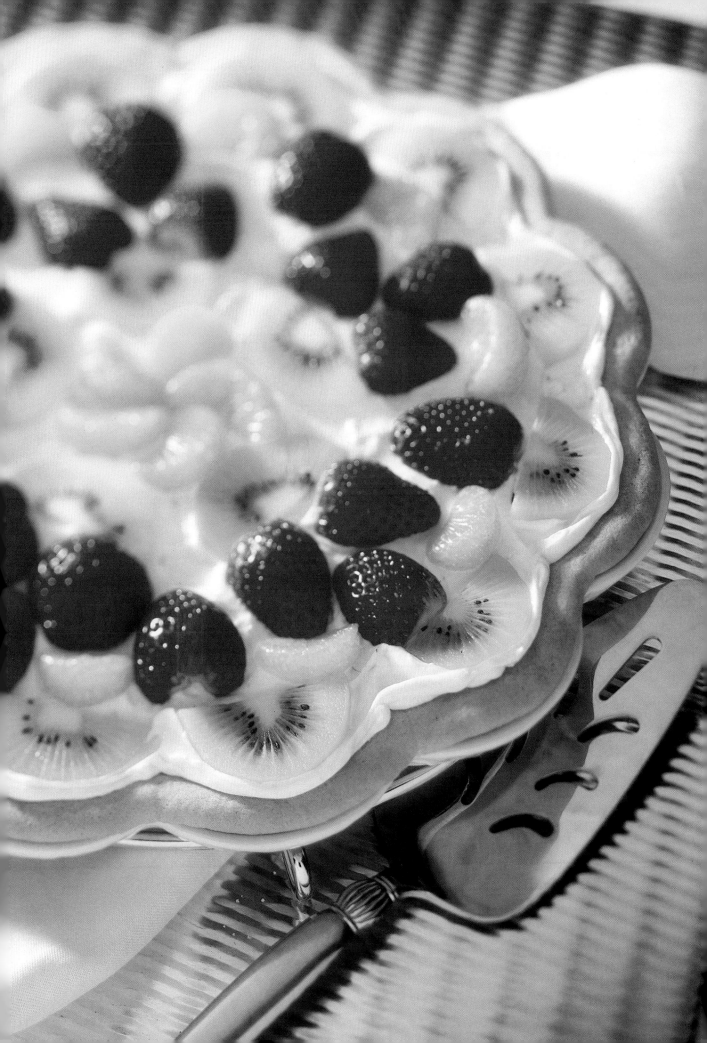

## Iced Cappuccino

**1 cup fat-free vanilla frozen yogurt or fat-free vanilla ice cream**
**1 cup cold strong-brewed coffee**
**1 teaspoon unsweetened cocoa powder**
**1 teaspoon vanilla**
**1 packet sugar substitute *or* equivalent of 2 teaspoons sugar**

**1.** Place all ingredients in food processor or blender; process until smooth. Place container in freezer; freeze 1½ to 2 hours or until top and sides of mixture are partially frozen.

**2.** Scrape sides of container; process until smooth and frothy. Garnish as desired. Serve immediately.                    *Makes 2 servings*

**Iced Mocha Cappuccino:** Increase amount of unsweetened cocoa powder to 1 tablespoon. Proceed as above.

### *N*utrients per Serving

| | | | | | |
|---|---|---|---|---|---|
| Calories | 105 | Saturated Fat | <1 g | Cholesterol | <1 mg |
| Calories from Fat | 0 % | Protein | 5 g | Sodium | 72 mg |
| Total Fat | <1 g | Carbohydrate | 21 g | Dietary Fiber | 0 g |

DIETARY EXCHANGES: 1½ Starch

*To add an extra flavor boost to this refreshing drink,*
*add orange peel, lemon peel or a dash of ground cinnamon*
*to your coffee grounds before brewing.*

*Iced Cappuccino*

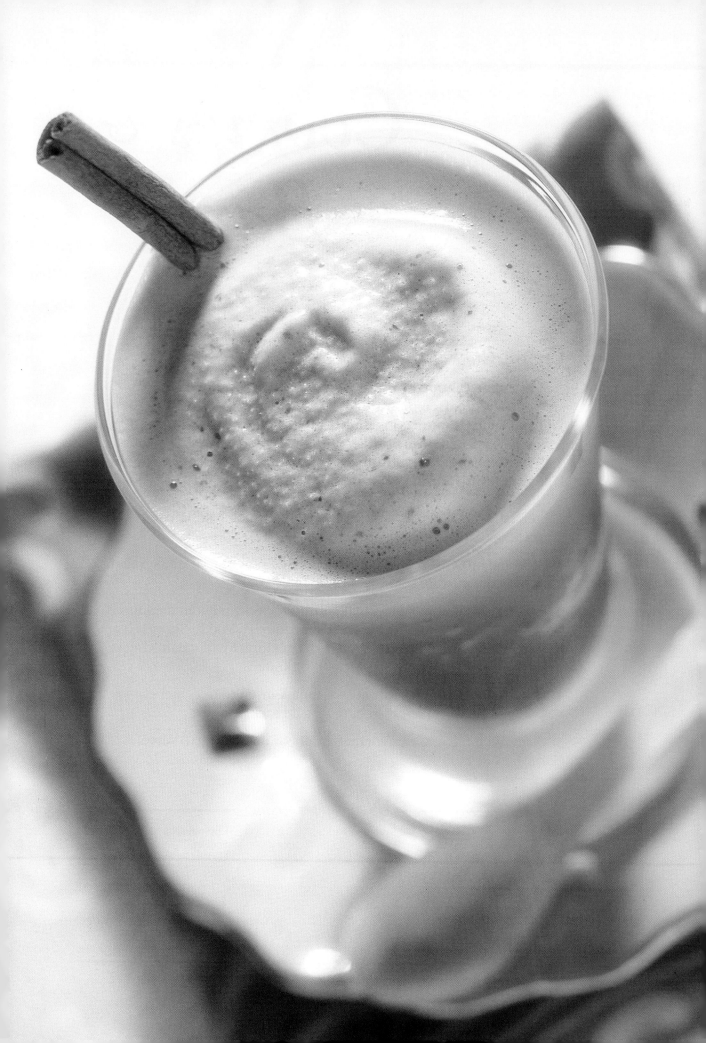

# Cookies & Bars

## Cream Cheese Brownie Royale

1 package (about 15 ounces) low-fat brownie mix
⅔ cup cold coffee or water
1 package (8 ounces) reduced-fat cream cheese, softened
¼ cup fat-free (skim) milk
5 packets sugar substitute *or* equivalent of 10 teaspoons sugar
½ teaspoon vanilla

**1.** Preheat oven to 350°F. Coat 13×9-inch nonstick baking pan with nonstick cooking spray; set aside.

**2.** Combine brownie mix and coffee in large bowl; stir until blended. Pour brownie mixture into prepared pan.

**3.** Beat cream cheese, milk, sugar substitute and vanilla in medium bowl with electric mixer at medium speed until smooth. Spoon cream cheese mixture in dollops over brownie mixture. Swirl cream cheese mixture into brownie mixture with tip of knife.

**4.** Bake 30 to 35 minutes or until toothpick inserted in center comes out clean. Cool completely in pan on wire rack.

**5.** Cover with foil and refrigerate 8 hours or until ready to serve. Garnish as desired.

*Makes 16 servings*

### Nutrients per Serving

| | | | | | |
|---|---|---|---|---|---|
| Calories | 143 | Saturated Fat | 2 g | Cholesterol | 7 mg |
| Calories from Fat | 26 % | Protein | 3 g | Sodium | 161 mg |
| Total Fat | 4 g | Carbohydrate | 23 g | Dietary Fiber | 1 g |

DIETARY EXCHANGES: 1½ Starch, ½ Fat

*Cream Cheese Brownie Royale*

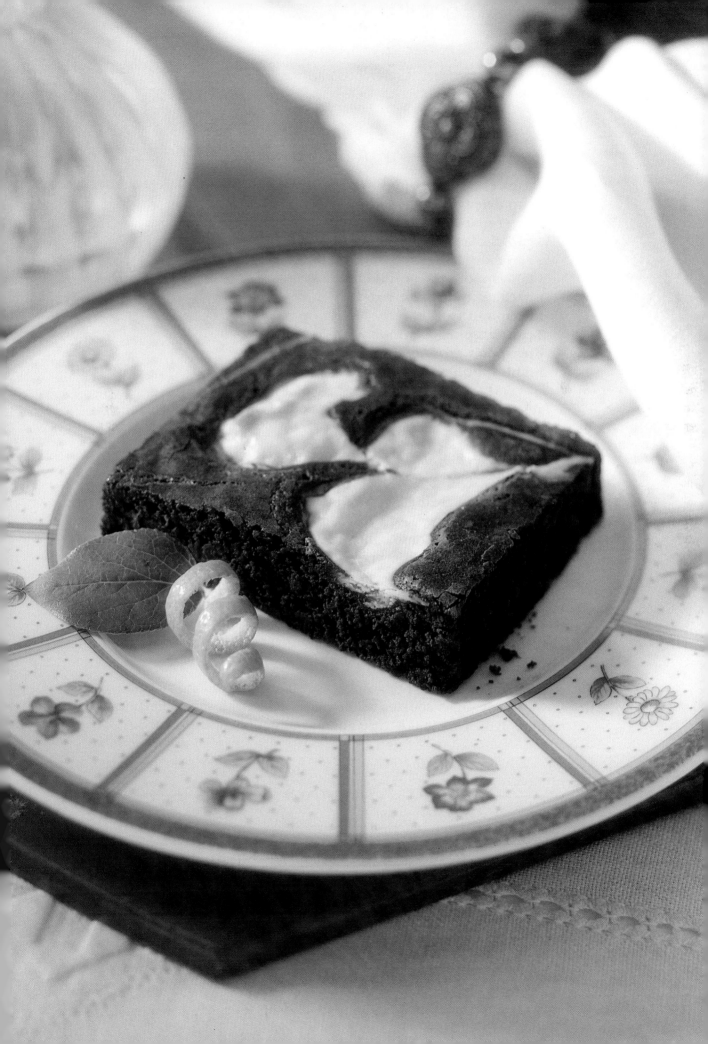

## Apple-Cranberry Crescent Cookies

1¼ cups chopped apples
½ cup dried cranberries
½ cup reduced-fat sour cream
¼ cup cholesterol-free egg substitute
¼ cup margarine or butter, melted
3 tablespoons sugar, divided
1 package quick-rise yeast
1 teaspoon vanilla
2 cups all-purpose flour
1 teaspoon ground cinnamon
1 tablespoon reduced-fat (2%) milk

**1.** Preheat oven to 350°F. Lightly coat cookie sheet with nonstick cooking spray; set aside.

**2.** Place apples and cranberries in food processor or blender; pulse to finely chop. Set aside.

**3.** Combine sour cream, egg substitute, margarine and 2 tablespoons sugar in medium bowl. Add yeast and vanilla. Add flour; stir to form ball. Turn dough out onto lightly floured work surface. Knead 1 minute. Cover with plastic wrap; allow to stand 10 minutes.

**4.** Divide dough into thirds. Roll one portion to 12-inch circle. Spread with ⅓ apple mixture (about ¼ cup). Cut dough to make 8 wedges. Roll up each wedge beginning at outside edge. Place on prepared cookie sheet; turn ends of cookies to form crescents. Repeat with remaining dough and apple mixture.

**5.** Combine remaining 1 tablespoon sugar and cinnamon in small bowl. Lightly brush cookies with milk; sprinkle with sugar-cinnamon mixture. Bake cookies 18 to 20 minutes or until lightly browned.

*Makes 24 servings*

### Nutrients per Serving

| | | | | | |
|---|---|---|---|---|---|
| Calories | 82 | Saturated Fat | 1 g | Cholesterol | 2 mg |
| Calories from Fat | 27% | Protein | 2 g | Sodium | 31 mg |
| Total Fat | 2 g | Carbohydrate | 13 g | Dietary Fiber | 1 g |

DIETARY EXCHANGES: 1 Starch

*Apple-Cranberry Crescent Cookies*

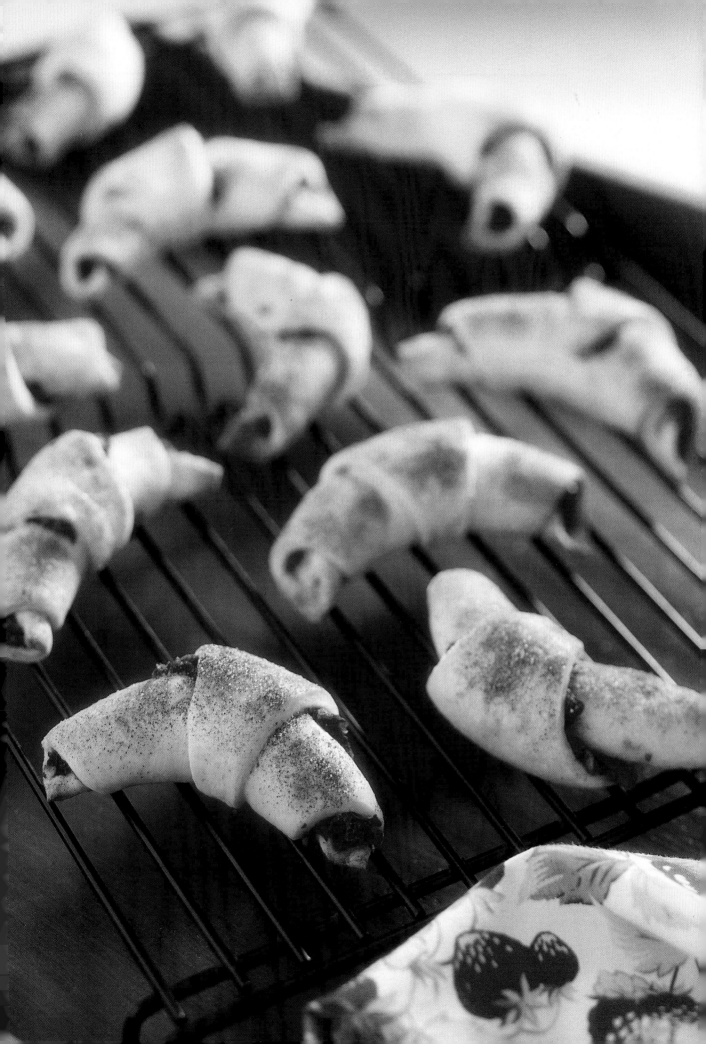

## Apricot Biscotti

**3 cups all-purpose flour**
**1½ teaspoons baking soda**
**½ teaspoon salt**
**3 eggs**
**⅔ cup sugar**
**1 teaspoon vanilla**
**½ cup chopped dried apricots***
**⅓ cup sliced almonds, chopped**
**1 tablespoon reduced-fat (2%) milk**

*Other chopped dried fruits, such as dried cherries, cranberries or blueberries, may be substituted.*

**1.** Preheat oven to 350°F. Lightly coat cookie sheet with nonstick cooking spray; set aside.

**2.** Combine flour, baking soda and salt in medium bowl; set aside.

**3.** Beat eggs, sugar and vanilla in large bowl with electric mixer at medium speed until combined. Add flour mixture; beat well.

**4.** Stir in apricots and almonds. Turn dough out onto lightly floured work surface. Knead 4 to 6 times. Roll dough into 20-inch log; place on prepared cookie sheet. Brush dough with milk.

**5.** Bake 30 minutes or until firm to touch. Remove from oven; cool 10 minutes. Diagonally slice into 30 biscotti. Place slices on cookie sheet. Bake 10 minutes; turn and bake an additional 10 minutes. Cool on wire racks. Store in airtight container. *Makes 30 servings*

### Nutrients per Serving

| | | | | | | |
|---|---|---|---|---|---|---|
| Calories | 86 | Saturated Fat | <1 g | Cholesterol | 21 mg |
| Calories from Fat | 13 % | Protein | 2 g | Sodium | 108 mg |
| Total Fat | 1 g | Carbohydrate | 16 g | Dietary Fiber | 1 g |

DIETARY EXCHANGES: 1 Starch

*Apricot Biscotti*

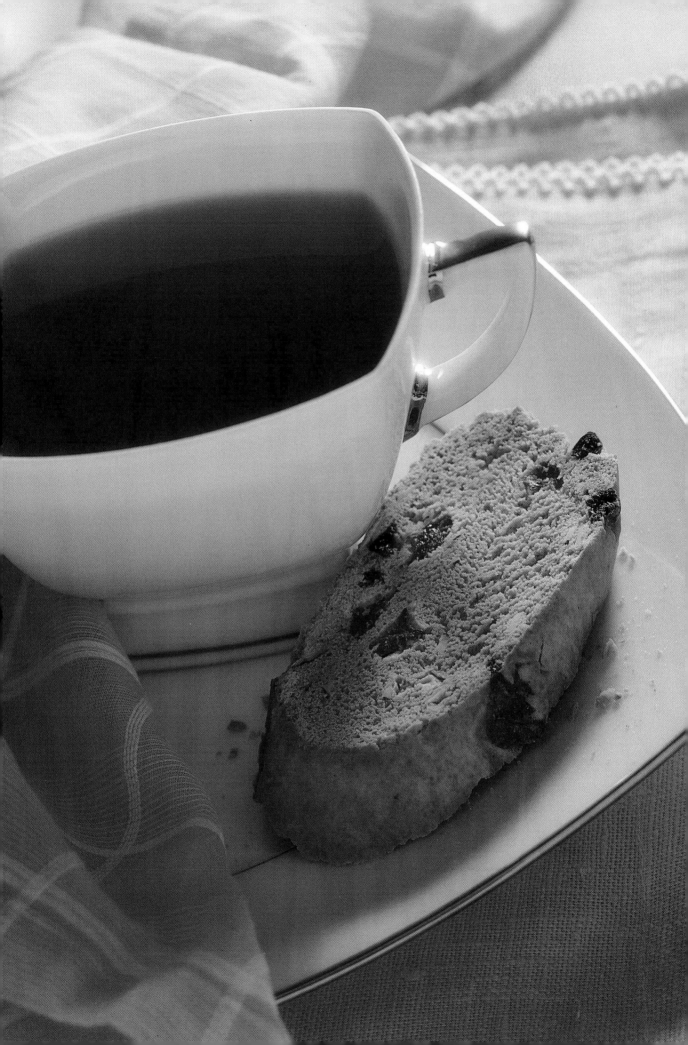

## Oatmeal-Date Cookies

½ cup packed light brown sugar
¼ cup margarine, softened
1 whole egg
1 egg white
1 tablespoon thawed frozen apple juice concentrate
1 teaspoon vanilla
1½ cups all-purpose flour
2 teaspoons baking soda
¼ teaspoon salt
1½ cups uncooked quick oats
½ cup chopped dates or raisins

**1.** Preheat oven to 350°F. Lightly coat cookie sheet with nonstick cooking spray; set aside.

**2.** Combine sugar and margarine in large bowl; mix well. Add egg, egg white, apple juice concentrate and vanilla; mix well.

**3.** Add flour, baking soda and salt; mix well. Stir in oats and dates. Drop dough by teaspoons onto prepared cookie sheet.

**4.** Bake 8 to 10 minutes or until edges are very lightly browned; center should still be soft.

**5.** Cool 1 minute on cookie sheet; remove to wire rack and cool completely.                    *Makes 36 servings*

### Nutrients per Serving

| | | | | | |
|---|---|---|---|---|---|
| Calories | 65 | Saturated Fat | <1 g | Cholesterol | 6 mg |
| Calories from Fat | 27 % | Protein | 1 g | Sodium | 106 mg |
| Total Fat | 2 g | Carbohydrate | 11 g | Dietary Fiber | 1 g |

DIETARY EXCHANGES: 1 Starch

*Oatmeal-Date Cookies*

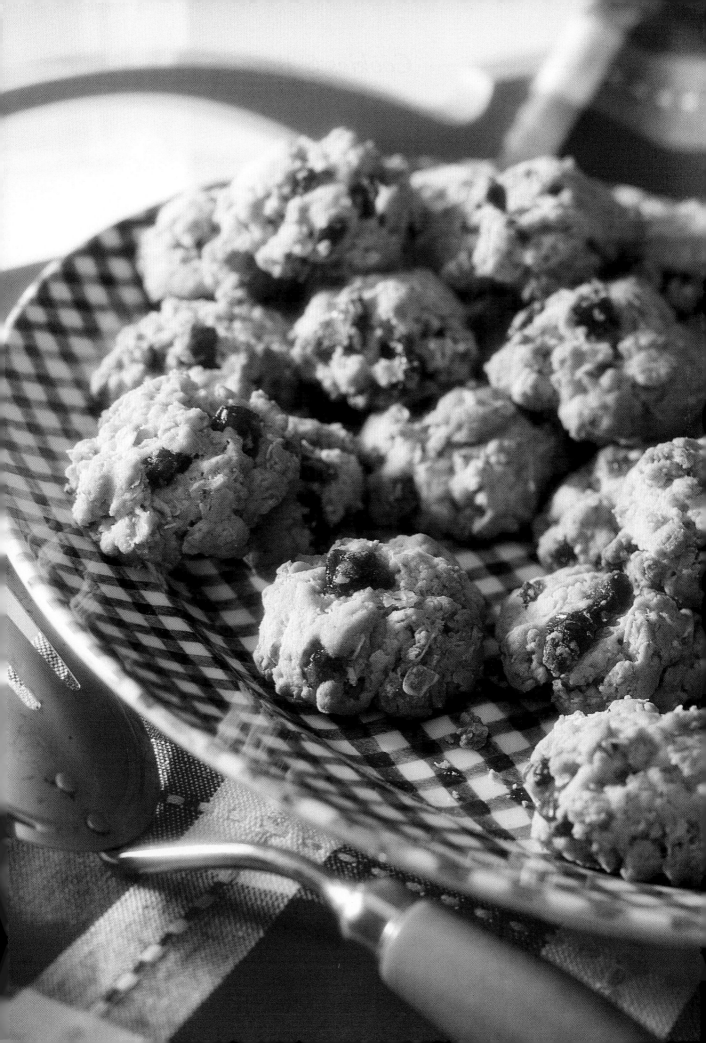

## Fig Bars

**DOUGH**
- ½ cup dried figs
- 6 tablespoons hot water
- 1 tablespoon sugar
- ⅔ cup all-purpose flour
- ½ cup uncooked quick oats
- ¾ teaspoon baking powder
- ¼ teaspoon salt
- 2 tablespoons oil
- 3 tablespoons fat-free (skim) milk

**ICING**
- 1 ounce reduced-fat cream cheese
- ⅓ cup powdered sugar
- ½ teaspoon vanilla

**1.** Preheat oven to 400°F. Lightly coat cookie sheet with nonstick cooking spray; set aside.

**2.** To prepare dough, combine figs, water and sugar in food processor or blender; process until figs are finely chopped. Set aside. Combine flour, oats, baking powder and salt in medium bowl. Add oil and just enough milk, 1 tablespoon at a time, until mixture forms a ball.

**3.** On lightly floured surface, roll dough into 12×9-inch rectangle. Place dough on prepared cookie sheet. Spread fig mixture in 2½-inch-wide strip lengthwise down center of rectangle. Make cuts almost to filling at ½-inch intervals on both 12-inch sides. Fold strips over filling, overlapping and crossing in center. Bake 15 to 18 minutes or until lightly browned.

**4.** To prepare icing, combine all ingredients in small bowl; mix well. Drizzle over braid. Cut into 12 pieces. *Makes 12 servings*

### Nutrients per Serving

| | | | | | |
|---|---|---|---|---|---|
| Calories | 104 | Saturated Fat | 1 g | Cholesterol | 1 mg |
| Calories from Fat | 26 % | Protein | 2 g | Sodium | 93 mg |
| Total Fat | 3 g | Carbohydrate | 18 g | Dietary Fiber | 1 g |

DIETARY EXCHANGES: 1 Starch, ½ Fat

## Peanut Butter Cereal Bars

3 cups miniature marshmallows
3 tablespoons margarine
½ cup reduced-fat peanut butter
3½ cups crisp rice cereal
1 cup uncooked quick oats
⅓ cup mini semisweet chocolate chips

**1.** Lightly coat 13×9-inch baking pan with nonstick cooking spray; set aside.

**2.** Combine marshmallows and margarine in large microwavable bowl. Microwave at HIGH 15 seconds; stir. Continue to microwave 1 minute; stir until marshmallows are melted and mixture is smooth. Add peanut butter; stir. Add cereal and oats; stir until well coated. Spread into prepared pan. Immediately sprinkle chocolate chips on top; lightly press.

**3.** Cool completely in pan. Cut into 40 bars.           *Makes 40 servings*

### Nutrients per Serving

| | | | | | |
|---|---|---|---|---|---|
| Calories | 65 | Saturated Fat | 1 g | Cholesterol | 0 mg |
| Calories from Fat | 41 % | Protein | 1 g | Sodium | 58 mg |
| Total Fat | 3 g | Carbohydrate | 10 g | Dietary Fiber | 1 g |

DIETARY EXCHANGES: ½ Starch, ½ Fat

*To make spreading the cereal mixture easier and cleanup a snap, lightly spray your spoon with nonstick cooking spray before stirring these bars.*

## Lemon-Cranberry Bars

½ **cup frozen lemonade concentrate, thawed**
½ **cup spoonable sugar substitute**
¼ **cup margarine**
1 **egg**
1½ **cups all-purpose flour**
2 **teaspoons grated lemon peel**
½ **teaspoon baking soda**
½ **teaspoon salt**
½ **cup dried cranberries**

**1.** Preheat oven to 375°F. Lightly coat 8-inch square baking pan with nonstick cooking spray; set aside.

**2.** Combine lemonade concentrate, sugar substitute, margarine and egg in medium bowl; mix well. Add flour, lemon peel, baking soda and salt; stir well. Stir in cranberries; pour into prepared pan.

**3.** Bake 20 minutes or until light brown. Cool completely in pan on wire rack. Cut into 16 squares. *Makes 16 servings*

*N*utrients per Serving

| Calories | 104 | Saturated Fat | 1 g | Cholesterol | 13 mg |
|---|---|---|---|---|---|
| Calories from Fat | 28 % | Protein | 3 g | Sodium | 150 mg |
| Total Fat | 3 g | Carbohydrate | 15 g | Dietary Fiber | <1 g |

DIETARY EXCHANGES: 1 Starch, ½ Fat

*Lemon-Cranberry Bars*

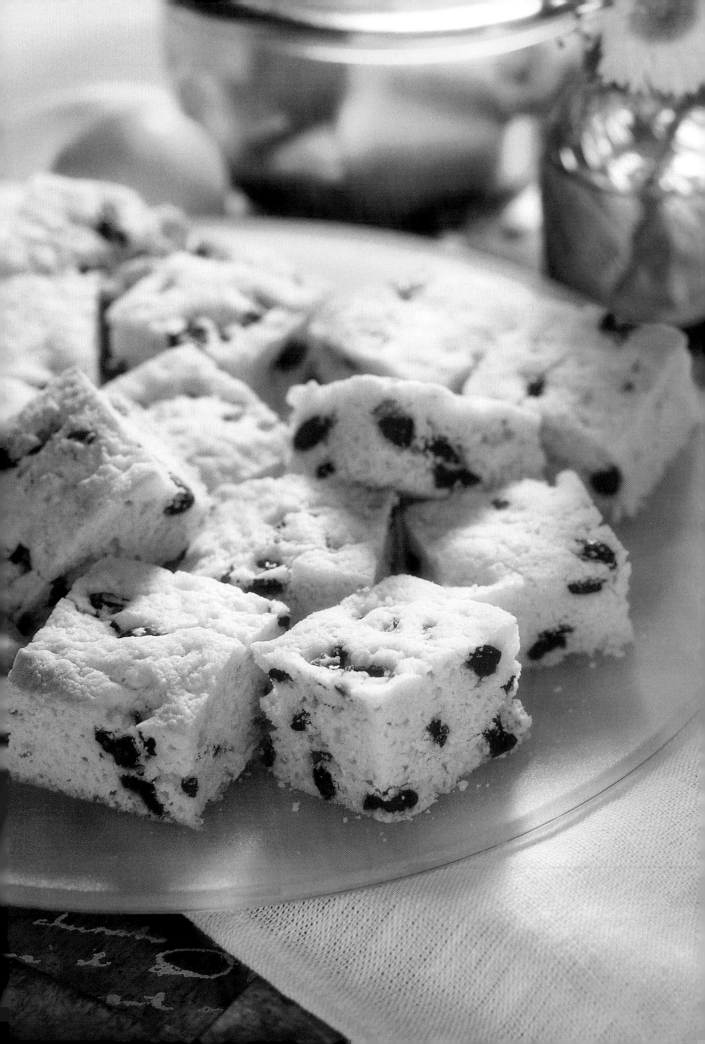

## Thumbprint Cookies

1½ cups all-purpose flour
1 teaspoon baking soda
¼ teaspoon salt
⅔ cup sugar
¼ cup margarine, softened
1 egg white
1 teaspoon vanilla
½ cup no-sugar-added raspberry or apricot fruit spread

**1.** Combine flour, baking soda and salt in medium bowl; set aside. Beat sugar, margarine, egg white and vanilla in large bowl with electric mixer at high speed until blended. Add flour mixture; mix well. Press mixture together to form a ball. Refrigerate ½ hour or overnight.

**2.** Preheat oven to 375°F. Lightly coat cookie sheet with nonstick cooking spray; set aside.

**3.** Shape dough into 1-inch balls with lightly floured hands; place on cookie sheet. Press down with thumb in center of each ball to form indention.

**4.** Bake 10 to 12 minutes or until golden brown. Remove to wire rack and cool completely. Fill each indention with about 1 teaspoon fruit spread.                    *Makes about 20 servings*

### Nutrients per Serving

| | | | | | | |
|---|---|---|---|---|---|---|
| Calories | 90 | Saturated Fat | <1 g | Cholesterol | 0 mg |
| Calories from Fat | 24 % | Protein | 1 g | Sodium | 130 mg |
| Total Fat | 2 g | Carbohydrate | 16 g | Dietary Fiber | <1 g |

DIETARY EXCHANGES: 1 Starch, ½ Fat

*Thumbprint Cookies*

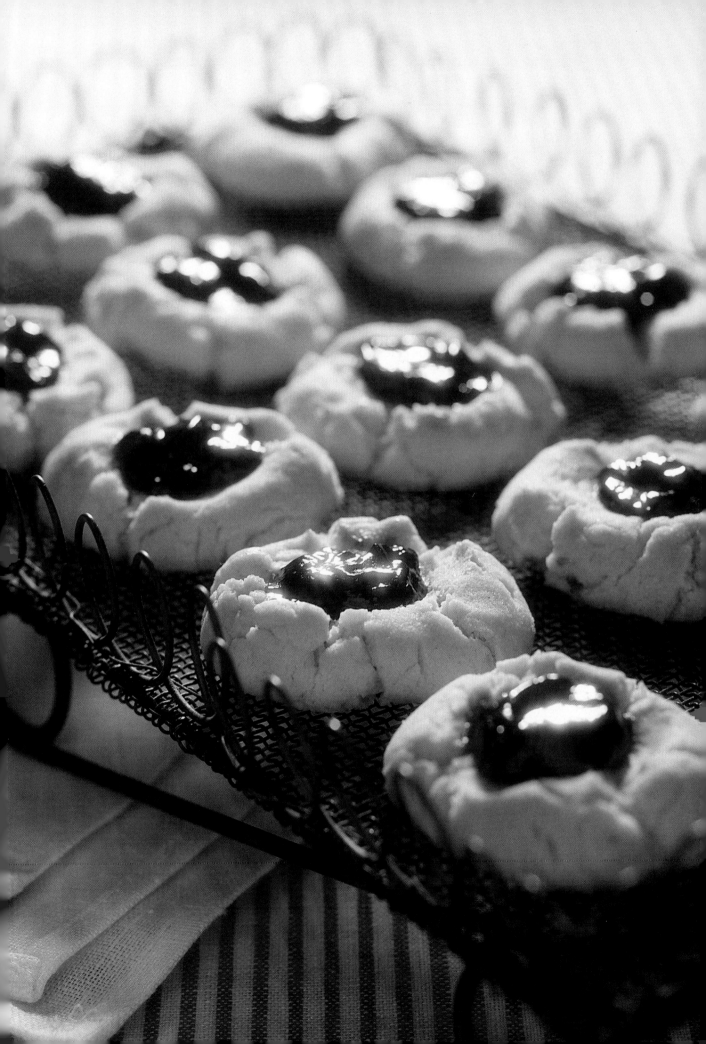

## Hikers' Bar Cookies

¾ cup all-purpose flour
½ cup packed brown sugar
½ cup uncooked quick oats
¼ cup toasted wheat germ
¼ cup unsweetened applesauce
¼ cup margarine or butter, softened
⅛ teaspoon salt
½ cup cholesterol-free egg substitute
¼ cup raisins
¼ cup dried cranberries
¼ cup sunflower kernels
1 tablespoon orange peel
1 teaspoon ground cinnamon

**1.** Preheat oven to 350°F. Lightly coat 13×9-inch baking pan with nonstick cooking spray; set aside.

**2.** Beat flour, sugar, oats, wheat germ, applesauce, margarine and salt in large bowl with electric mixer at medium speed until well blended. Add egg substitute, raisins, cranberries, sunflower kernels, orange peel and cinnamon. Spread into pan.

**3.** Bake 15 minutes or until firm to touch. Cool completely in pan on wire rack. Cut into 24 squares. *Makes 24 servings*

### Nutrients per Serving

| | | | | | |
|---|---|---|---|---|---|
| Calories | 80 | Saturated Fat | <1 g | Cholesterol | 0 mg |
| Calories from Fat | 33 % | Protein | 2 g | Sodium | 46 mg |
| Total Fat | 3 g | Carbohydrate | 12 g | Dietary Fiber | 1 g |

DIETARY EXCHANGES: 1 Starch, ½ Fat

*Hikers' Bar Cookies*

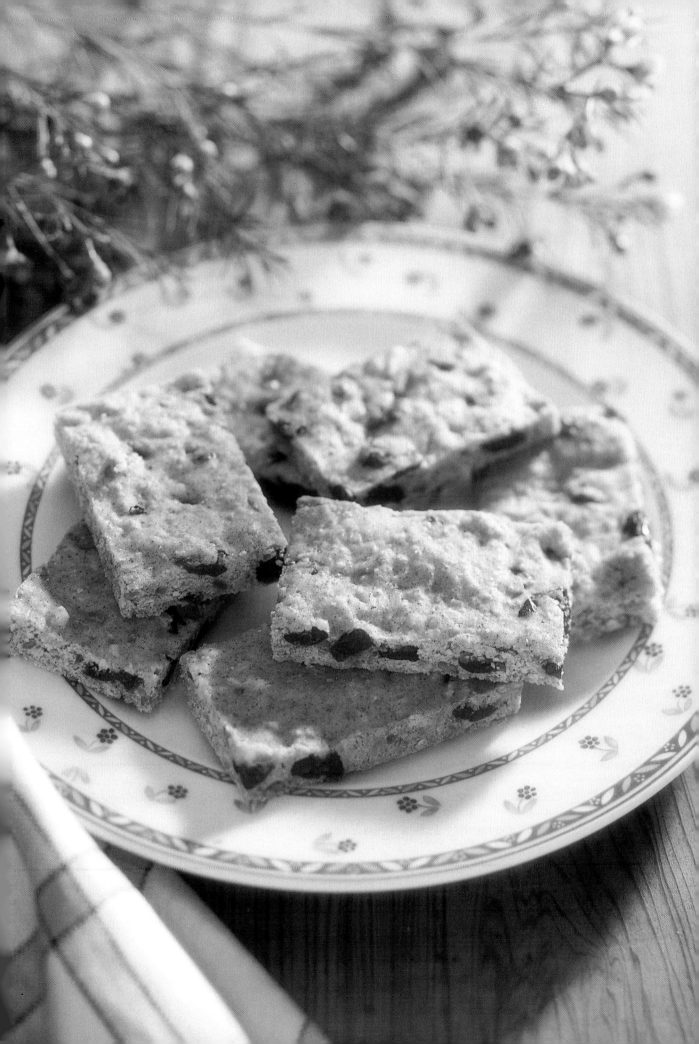

# Cakes & Cheesecakes

## Cherry Bowl Cheesecakes

**1 package (8 ounces) fat-free cream cheese, softened**
**1 package (8 ounces) reduced-fat cream cheese, softened**
**2 tablespoons fat-free (skim) milk**
**4 packets sugar substitute *or* equivalent of 8 teaspoons sugar**
**¼ teaspoon almond extract**
**40 reduced-fat vanilla wafers**
**1 can (16 ounces) light cherry pie filling**

**1.** Beat cream cheese, milk, sugar substitute and almond extract in medium bowl with electric mixer at high speed until well blended.

**2.** Place one vanilla wafer on bottom of 4-ounce ramekin.* Arrange four additional vanilla wafers around side of ramekin. Repeat with remaining wafers. Fill each ramekin with ¼ cup cream cheese mixture; top each with ¼ cup cherry pie filling. Cover with plastic wrap; refrigerate 8 hours or overnight.                          *Makes 8 servings*

*\*Note: If ramekins are not available, you may substitute with custard dishes or line 8 muffin cups with paper liners and fill according to above directions.*

### Nutrients per Serving

| | | | | | |
|---|---|---|---|---|---|
| Calories | 214 | Saturated Fat | 4 g | Cholesterol | 16 mg |
| Calories from Fat | 29 % | Protein | 9 g | Sodium | 387 mg |
| Total Fat | 7 g | Carbohydrate | 29 g | Dietary Fiber | 1 g |

DIETARY EXCHANGES: 1 Starch, 1 Fruit, 1½ Fat

*Cherry Bowl Cheesecake*

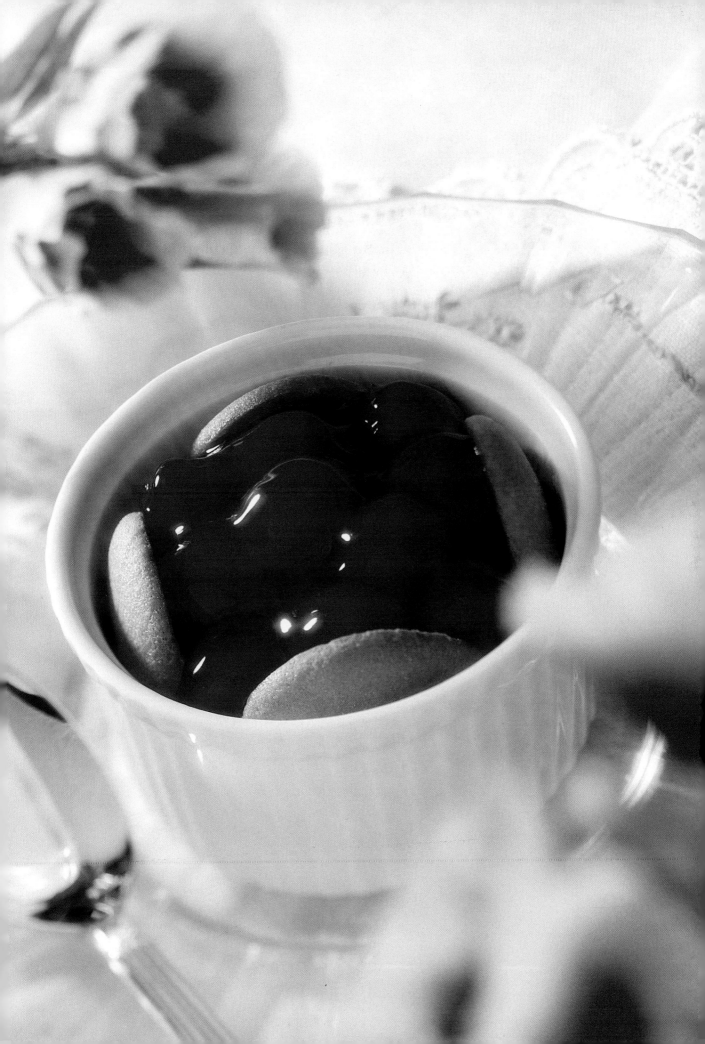

## Chocolate Bundt Cake with White Chocolate Glaze

**CAKE**
>  1 package (18.25 ounces) chocolate cake mix
>  3 whole eggs *or* ¾ cup cholesterol-free egg substitute
>  3 jars (2½ ounces each) puréed baby food prunes
>  ¾ cup warm water
>  2 to 3 teaspoons instant coffee granules
>  2 tablespoons canola oil

**GLAZE**
>  ½ cup white chocolate chips
>  1 tablespoon milk

**1.** Preheat oven to 350°F. Lightly grease and flour Bundt pan; set aside.

**2.** Beat all ingredients for Bundt cake in large bowl with electric mixer at high speed 2 minutes. Pour into prepared pan. Bake 40 minutes or until toothpick inserted in center comes out clean; cool 10 minutes. Invert cake onto serving plate; cool completely.

**3.** To prepare glaze, combine white chocolate chips and milk in small microwavable bowl. Microwave at MEDIUM (50% power) 50 seconds; stir. Microwave at MEDIUM at additional 30-second intervals until chips are completely melted; stir well after each 30 second interval.

**4.** Pour warm glaze over cooled cake. Let stand about 30 minutes. Garnish as desired; serve. *Makes 16 servings*

---

### Nutrients per Serving

| | | | | | |
|---|---|---|---|---|---|
| Calories | 209 | Saturated Fat | 3 g | Cholesterol | 41 mg |
| Calories from Fat | 33 % | Protein | 3 g | Sodium | 259 mg |
| Total Fat | 8 g | Carbohydrate | 32 g | Dietary Fiber | 1 g |

DIETARY EXCHANGES: 2 Starch, 1½ Fat

*Chocolate Bundt Cake with White Chocolate Glaze*

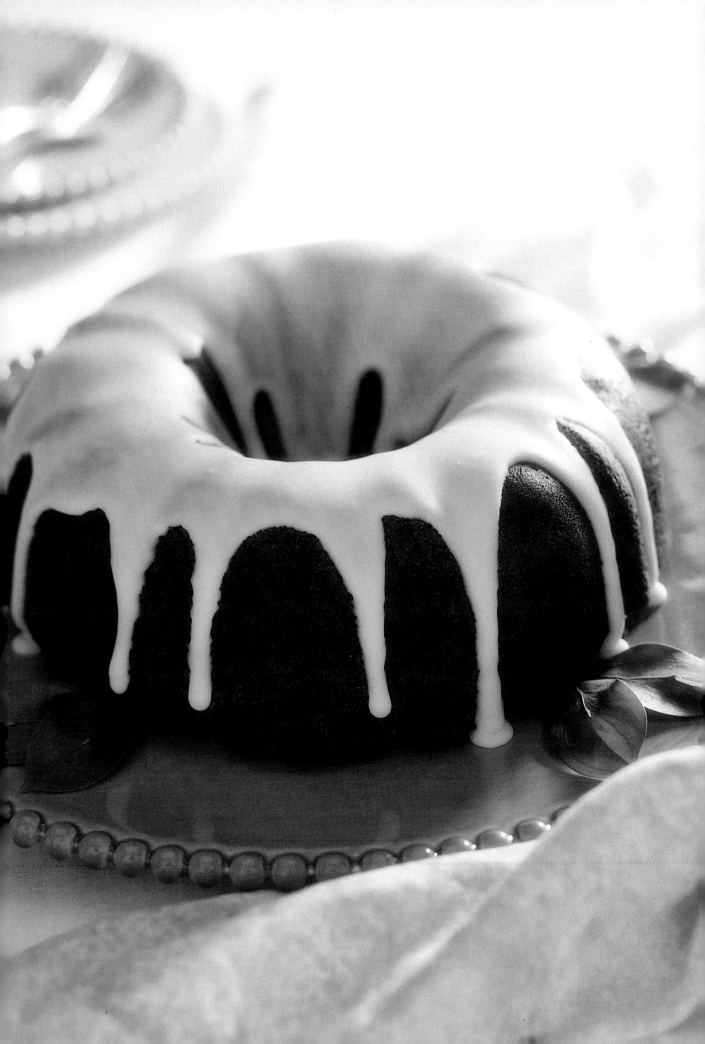

## New-Fashioned Gingerbread Cake

  **2 cups cake flour**
  **1 teaspoon baking powder**
  **1 teaspoon ground ginger**
  **½ teaspoon baking soda**
  **½ teaspoon ground cinnamon**
  **½ teaspoon ground nutmeg**
  **¼ teaspoon ground cloves**
  **¾ cup water**
  **⅓ cup packed brown sugar**
  **¼ cup molasses**
  **3 tablespoons canola oil**
  **2 tablespoons finely minced crystallized ginger (optional)**
  **2 tablespoons powdered sugar**

**1.** Preheat oven to 350°F. Coat 8-inch square baking pan with nonstick cooking spray; set aside.

**2.** Combine flour, baking powder, ginger, baking soda, cinnamon, nutmeg and cloves in large bowl; mix well.

**3.** Beat water, brown sugar, molasses and oil in small bowl with electric mixer at low speed until well blended. Pour into flour mixture; beat until just blended. Stir in crystallized ginger.

**4.** Pour into prepared pan. Bake 30 to 35 minutes or until toothpick inserted in center comes out clean. Let cool 10 minutes. Sprinkle with powdered sugar just before serving.                    *Makes 9 servings*

### Nutrients per Serving

| Calories | 188 | Saturated Fat | <1 g | Cholesterol | 0 mg |
|---|---|---|---|---|---|
| Calories from Fat | 23 % | Protein | 2 g | Sodium | 133 mg |
| Total Fat | 5 g | Carbohydrate | 34 g | Dietary Fiber | 1 g |

DIETARY EXCHANGES: 2 Starch, 1 Fat

## Chocolate Pudding Cake

**CAKE**

    1 cup all-purpose flour
    ⅓ cup sugar
    10 packets sugar substitute *or* equivalent of 20 teaspoons sugar
    3 tablespoons unsweetened cocoa
    2 teaspoons baking powder
    ½ teaspoon salt
    2 tablespoons canola oil
    2 teaspoons vanilla

**SAUCE**

    ¼ cup sugar
    10 packets sugar substitute *or* equivalent of 20 teaspoons sugar
    3 tablespoons unsweetened cocoa
    1¾ cups boiling water

**1.** Preheat oven to 350°F. Combine all cake ingredients in large bowl; mix well. Pour into ungreased 9-inch square baking pan.

**2.** To prepare sauce, sprinkle ¼ cup sugar, 10 packets sugar substitute and 3 tablespoons cocoa over batter in pan. Pour boiling water over top. *(Do not stir.)*

**3.** Bake 40 minutes or until cake portion has risen to top of pan and sauce is bubbling underneath. Serve immediately.    *Makes 9 servings*

---

### Nutrients per Serving

| | | | | | |
|---|---|---|---|---|---|
| Calories | 145 | Saturated Fat | <1 g | Cholesterol | <1 mg |
| Calories from Fat | 20 % | Protein | 4 g | Sodium | 245 mg |
| Total Fat | 3 g | Carbohydrate | 25 g | Dietary Fiber | <1 g |

DIETARY EXCHANGES: 1½ Starch, ½ Fat

## Luscious Lime Angel Food Cake Rolls

**1 package (16 ounces) angel food cake mix**
**2 cartons (8 ounces each) lime-flavored nonfat yogurt with**
    **aspartame sweetener**
**2 drops green food coloring (optional)**
    **Lime slices (optional)**

**1.** Preheat oven to 350°F. Line two 17×11¼×1-inch jelly roll pans with parchment or waxed paper; set aside.

**2.** Prepare angel food cake batter according to package directions. Divide batter evenly between prepared pans. Draw knife through batter to remove large air bubbles. Bake 12 minutes or until cakes are lightly browned and toothpick inserted in centers comes out clean.

**3.** Invert each cake onto separate clean towel. Starting at short end, roll warm cake, jelly-roll fashion with towel inside. Cool cakes completely.

**4.** Place 1 to 2 drops green food coloring in each carton of yogurt; stir well. Unroll cake; remove towel. Spread each cake with 1 carton yogurt, leaving 1-inch border. Roll up cake; place seam side down. Slice each cake roll into 8 pieces. Garnish with lime slices. Refrigerate if not serving immediately.
*Makes 16 servings*

### Nutrients per Serving

| | | | | | |
|---|---|---|---|---|---|
| Calories | 136 | Saturated Fat | <1 g | Cholesterol | 0 mg |
| Calories from Fat | 1 % | Protein | 4 g | Sodium | 252 mg |
| Total Fat | <1 g | Carbohydrate | 30 g | Dietary Fiber | <1 g |

DIETARY EXCHANGES: 2 Starch

*Luscious Lime Angel Food Cake Roll*

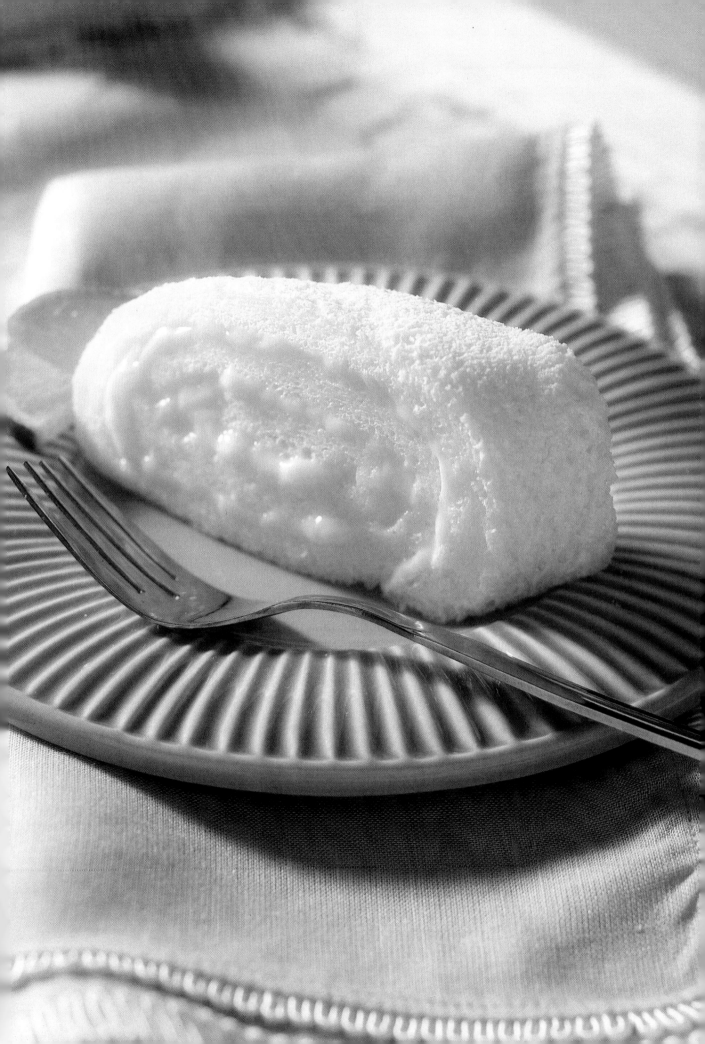

## Ginger-Crusted Pumpkin Cheesecake

12 whole low-fat honey graham crackers, broken into pieces
3 tablespoons reduced-fat margarine, melted
½ teaspoon ground ginger
1 can (15 ounces) solid-pack pumpkin
2 packages (8 ounces each) fat-free cream cheese, softened
1 package (8 ounces) reduced-fat cream cheese, softened
1 cup sugar
1 cup cholesterol-free egg substitute
½ cup nonfat evaporated milk
1 tablespoon vanilla
1 teaspoon ground cinnamon
½ teaspoon ground nutmeg
¼ teaspoon salt
2 cups thawed frozen reduced-fat whipped topping
    Additional ground nutmeg (optional)

**1.** Preheat oven 350°F. Coat 9-inch springform baking pan with nonstick cooking spray; set aside.

**2.** Place graham crackers, margarine and ginger in food processor or blender; pulse until coarse in texture. Gently press crumb mixture onto bottom and ¾ inch up side of pan. Bake 10 minutes or until lightly browned; cool slightly on wire rack.

**3.** Beat remaining ingredients except whipped topping and additional nutmeg in large bowl with electric mixer at medium-high speed until smooth; pour into pie crust. Bake 1 hour and 15 minutes or until top begins to crack and center moves very little when pan is shaken back and forth. Cool on wire rack to room temperature; refrigerate until ready to serve.

**4.** Just before serving, spoon 1 tablespoon whipped topping on each serving; sprinkle lightly with additional nutmeg.     *Makes 16 servings*

### Nutrients per Serving

| | | | | | |
|---|---|---|---|---|---|
| Calories | 187 | Saturated Fat | 4 g | Cholesterol | 9 mg |
| Calories from Fat | 32 % | Protein | 8 g | Sodium | 338 mg |
| Total Fat | 6 g | Carbohydrate | 23 g | Dietary Fiber | 1 g |

DIETARY EXCHANGES: 1½ Starch, 1 Lean Meat, ½ Fat

*Ginger-Crusted Pumpkin Cheesecake*

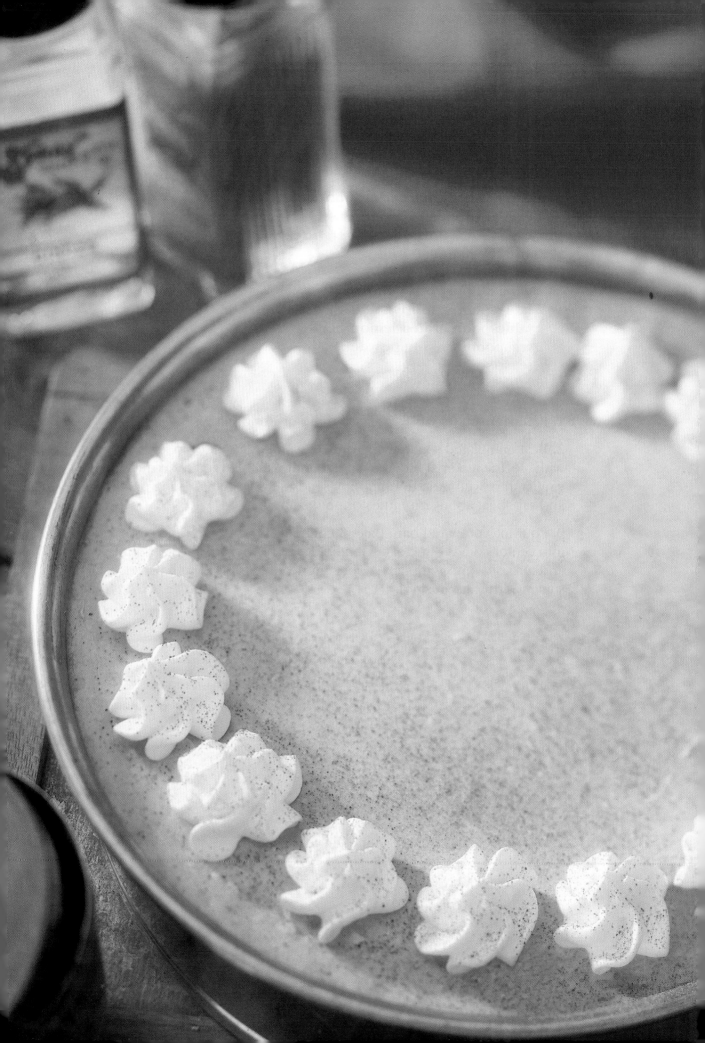

## Lemon Poppy Seed Bundt Cake

  1 cup granulated sugar
  ½ cup (1 stick) margarine, softened
  1 egg, at room temperature
  2 egg whites, at room temperature
  ¾ cup low-fat (1%) milk
  2 teaspoons vanilla
  2 cups all-purpose flour
  2 tablespoons poppy seeds
  1 tablespoon grated lemon peel
  2 teaspoons baking powder
  ¼ teaspoon salt
  1½ tablespoons powdered sugar

**1.** Preheat oven to 350°F. Grease and flour Bundt pan; set aside.

**2.** Beat granulated sugar, margarine, egg and egg whites in large bowl with electric mixer at medium speed until well blended. Add milk and vanilla; mix well. Add flour, poppy seeds, lemon peel, baking powder and salt; beat about 2 minutes or until smooth.

**3.** Pour into prepared pan. Bake 30 minutes or until toothpick inserted into center comes out clean. Gently loosen cake from pan with knife and turn out onto wire rack; cool completely. Sprinkle with powdered sugar. Garnish as desired. *Makes 16 servings*

### Nutrients per Serving

| | | | | | |
|---|---|---|---|---|---|
| Calories | 178 | Saturated Fat | 1 g | Cholesterol | 14 mg |
| Calories from Fat | 34 % | Protein | 3 g | Sodium | 181 mg |
| Total Fat | 7 g | Carbohydrate | 26 g | Dietary Fiber | 1 g |

DIETARY EXCHANGES: 1½ Starch, 1½ Fat

*Lemon Poppy Seed Bundt Cake*

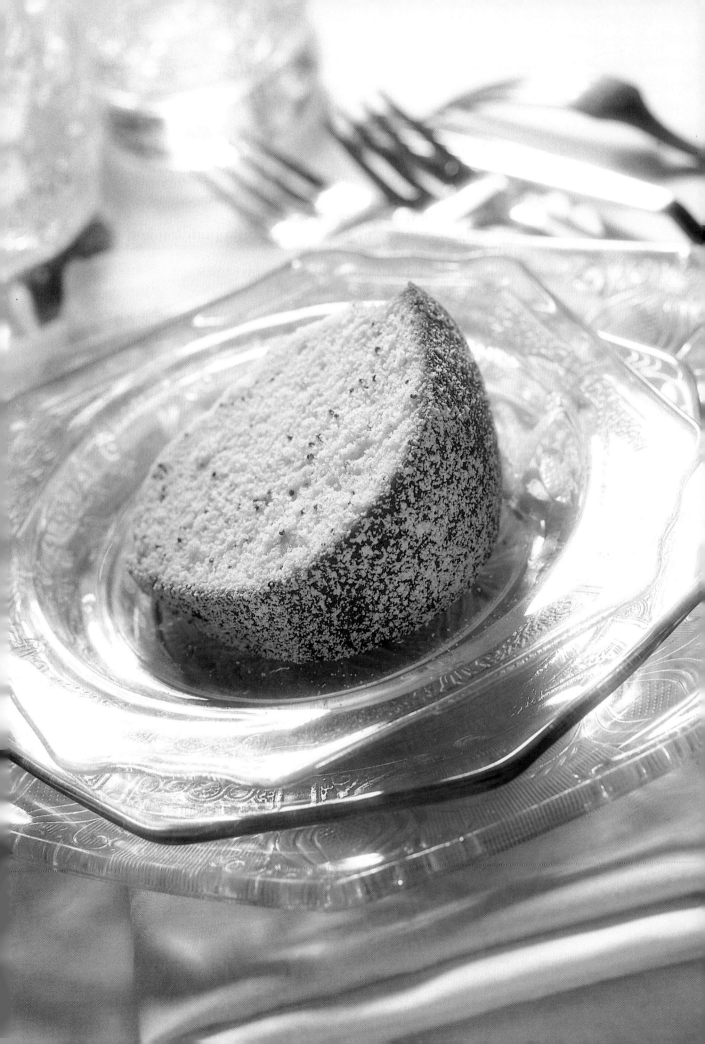

## *Boston Babies*

  1 package (18.25 ounces) yellow cake mix
  3 eggs *or* ¾ cup cholesterol-free egg substitute
  ⅓ cup unsweetened applesauce
  1 package (4 serving size) sugar-free vanilla pudding and pie
      filling mix
  2 cups low-fat (1%) milk or fat-free (skim) milk
  ⅓ cup sugar
  ⅓ cup unsweetened cocoa powder
  1 tablespoon cornstarch
1½ cups water
1½ teaspoons vanilla

**1.** Line 24 (2½-inch) muffin cups with paper liners; set aside.

**2.** Prepare cake mix according to lower fat package directions, using 3 eggs and applesauce. Pour batter into prepared muffin cups. Bake according to package directions; cool completely. Freeze 12 cupcakes for future use.

**3.** Prepare pudding according to package directions, using 2 cups milk; cover and refrigerate.

**4.** Combine sugar, cocoa, cornstarch and water in large microwavable bowl; whisk until smooth. Microwave at HIGH 4 to 6 minutes, stirring every 2 minutes, until slightly thickened. Stir in vanilla.

**5.** To serve, drizzle 2 tablespoons chocolate glaze over each dessert plate. Cut cupcakes in half; place 2 halves on top of chocolate on each dessert plate. Top each with about 2 heaping tablespoonfuls pudding. Garnish with pineapple halves and orange peel. Serve immediately.

*Makes 12 servings*

### *Nutrients per Serving*

| | | | | | |
|---|---|---|---|---|---|
| Calories | 158 | Saturated Fat | 1 g | Cholesterol | 29 mg |
| Calories from Fat | 22 % | Protein | 3 g | Sodium | 175 mg |
| Total Fat | 4 g | Carbohydrate | 28 g | Dietary Fiber | <1 g |

DIETARY EXCHANGES: 2 Starch, ½ Fat

*Boston Baby*

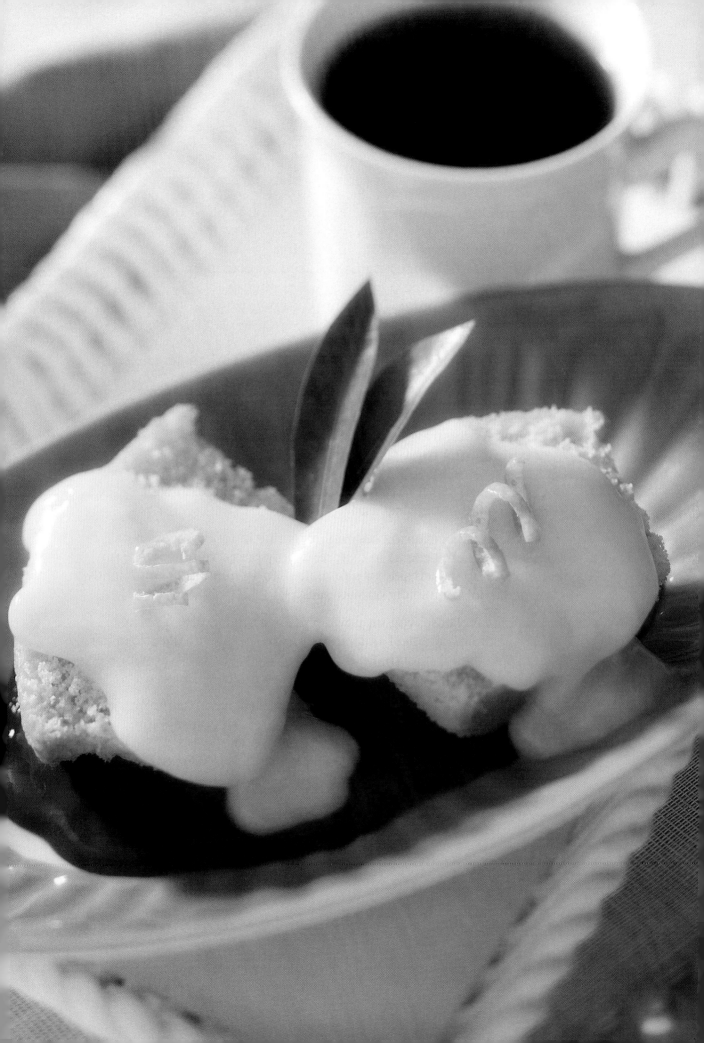

## Key Lime Cheesecake with Strawberries and Fresh Mint

**12 whole low-fat honey graham crackers, broken into small
  pieces
2 tablespoons reduced-fat margarine
2 packages (8 ounces each) reduced-fat cream cheese
1 package (8 ounces) fat-free cream cheese
1 container (8 ounces) nonfat plain yogurt
⅔ cup powdered sugar
¼ cup lime juice
8 packets sugar substitute *or* equivalent of ⅓ cup sugar,
  divided
2 teaspoons lime peel
1½ teaspoons vanilla
3 cups fresh strawberries, quartered
2 tablespoons finely chopped mint leaves**

**1.** Preheat oven 350°F. Coat 9-inch springform baking pan with nonstick cooking spray; set aside.

**2.** Place graham cracker pieces and margarine in food processor or blender; pulse until coarse in texture. Gently press crumb mixture on bottom and up ½ inch side of pan. Bake 8 to 10 minutes or until lightly browned; cool completely on wire rack.

**3.** Beat cream cheese, yogurt, powdered sugar, lime juice, 6 packets sugar substitute, lime peel and vanilla in large bowl with electric mixer at high speed until smooth. Pour into cooled pie crust. Cover with plastic wrap; freeze 2 hours or refrigerate overnight.

**4.** Combine strawberries, remaining 2 packets sugar substitute and mint in medium bowl 30 minutes before serving; set aside. Just before serving, spoon strawberry mixture over cheesecake.

*Makes 12 servings*

### Nutrients per Serving

| | | | | | | |
|---|---|---|---|---|---|---|
| Calories | 176 | Saturated Fat | 5 g | Cholesterol | 20 mg |
| Calories from Fat | 39 % | Protein | 8 g | Sodium | 341 mg |
| Total Fat | 7 g | Carbohydrate | 18 g | Dietary Fiber | 1 g |

DIETARY EXCHANGES: 1 Starch, 1 Lean Meat, 1 Fat

*Key Lime Cheesecake with Strawberries and Fresh Mint*

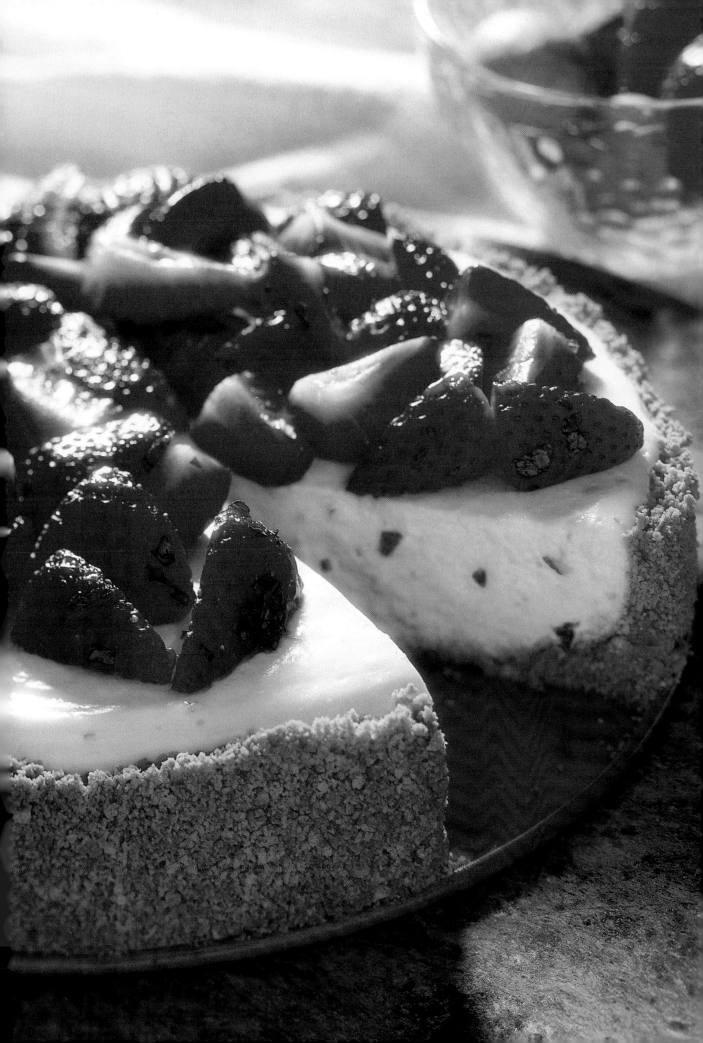

# Pies & Such

## Frozen Sundae Pie

**26 chocolate wafer cookies**
**4 cups fat-free ice cream, slightly softened**
**2 tablespoons fat-free hot fudge ice cream topping**
**1 cup banana slices**
**2 tablespoons fat-free caramel ice cream topping**
**1 ounce reduced-fat dry roasted peanuts, crushed**

**1.** Place cookies on bottom and around side of 9-inch pie pan. Carefully spoon ice cream into pie pan; cover with plastic wrap. Freeze 2 hours or overnight or until firm.

**2.** Just before serving, place fudge topping in small microwavable bowl; microwave at HIGH 10 seconds. Drizzle pie with fudge topping; top with banana slices. Place caramel topping in small microwavable bowl; microwave at HIGH 10 seconds. Drizzle over bananas; sprinkle with peanuts. *Makes 8 servings*

**Note:** If desired, the pie may be assembled the night before without the bananas. Top pie with bananas at time of serving.

### Nutrients per Serving

| | | | | | |
|---|---|---|---|---|---|
| Calories | 252 | Saturated Fat | 1 g | Cholesterol | <1 mg |
| Calories from Fat | 16 % | Protein | 7 g | Sodium | 210 mg |
| Total Fat | 5 g | Carbohydrate | 49 g | Dietary Fiber | 1 g |

DIETARY EXCHANGES: 3 Starch, 1 Fat

*Frozen Sundae Pie*

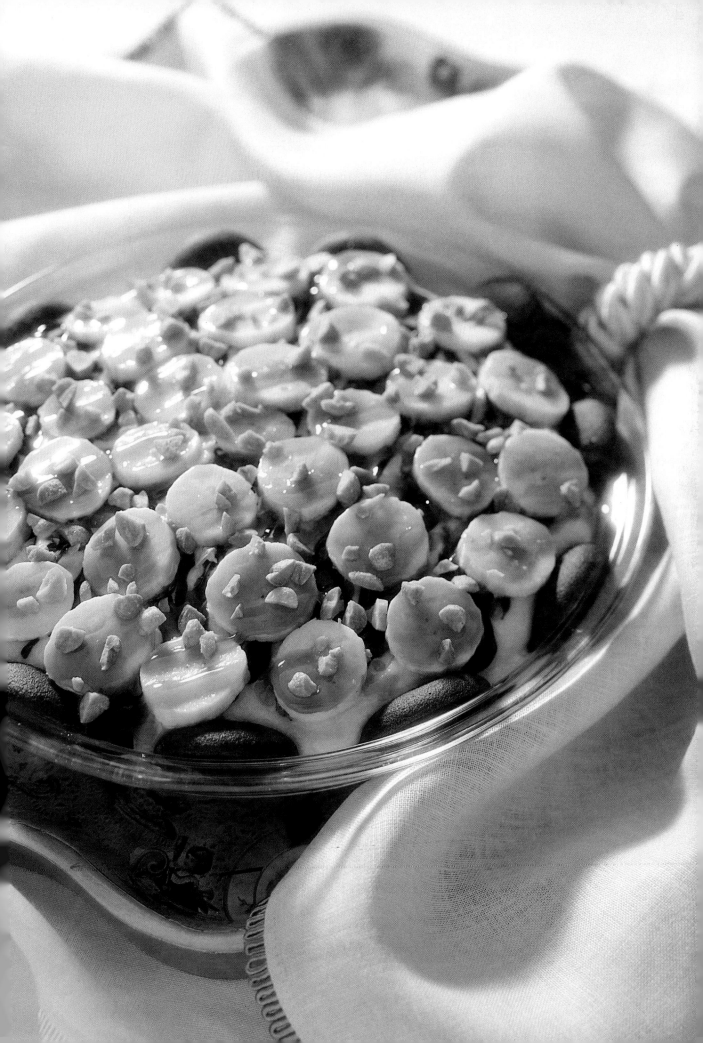

## Provençal Apple-Walnut Crumb Pie

**5 cups peeled and thinly sliced Red Delicious apples**
**1 tablespoon lemon juice**
**¾ teaspoon vanilla**
**½ cup packed dark brown sugar**
**⅓ cup plus 3 tablespoons all-purpose flour, divided**
**1 teaspoon ground cinnamon**
**¼ teaspoon ground nutmeg**
**1 frozen reduced-fat pie crust**
**¼ cup chopped walnuts**
**2 tablespoons granulated sugar**
**2 tablespoons cold margarine, cut into small pieces**

**1.** Preheat oven 425°F. Place baking sheet in oven while preheating.

**2.** Combine, apples, lemon juice and vanilla in large bowl; set aside.

**3.** Combine brown sugar, 3 tablespoons flour, cinnamon and nutmeg in medium bowl; blend thoroughly. Add brown sugar mixture to apple mixture; toss to coat. Spoon into pie crust; set aside.

**4.** Heat 10-inch nonstick skillet over medium-high heat until very hot. Add nuts; cook 2 minutes, stirring constantly with wooden spoon until lightly browned and fragrant. Remove from heat; set aside.

**5.** Combine remaining ⅓ cup flour and granulated sugar in small bowl. Cut in margarine using pastry blender or two knives until mixture resembles course crumbs; sprinkle evenly over pie. Top with walnuts.

**6.** Bake 35 to 40 minutes or until bubbly and apples are tender in center.

*Makes 8 servings*

### Nutrients per Serving

| | | | | | | |
|---|---|---|---|---|---|---|
| Calories | 292 | Saturated Fat | 2 g | Cholesterol | 0 mg |
| Calories from Fat | 33 % | Protein | 3 g | Sodium | 135 mg |
| Total Fat | 11 g | Carbohydrate | 49 g | Dietary Fiber | 3 g |

DIETARY EXCHANGES: 2 Starch, 1 Fruit, 2 Fat

*Provençal Apple-Walnut Crumb Pie*

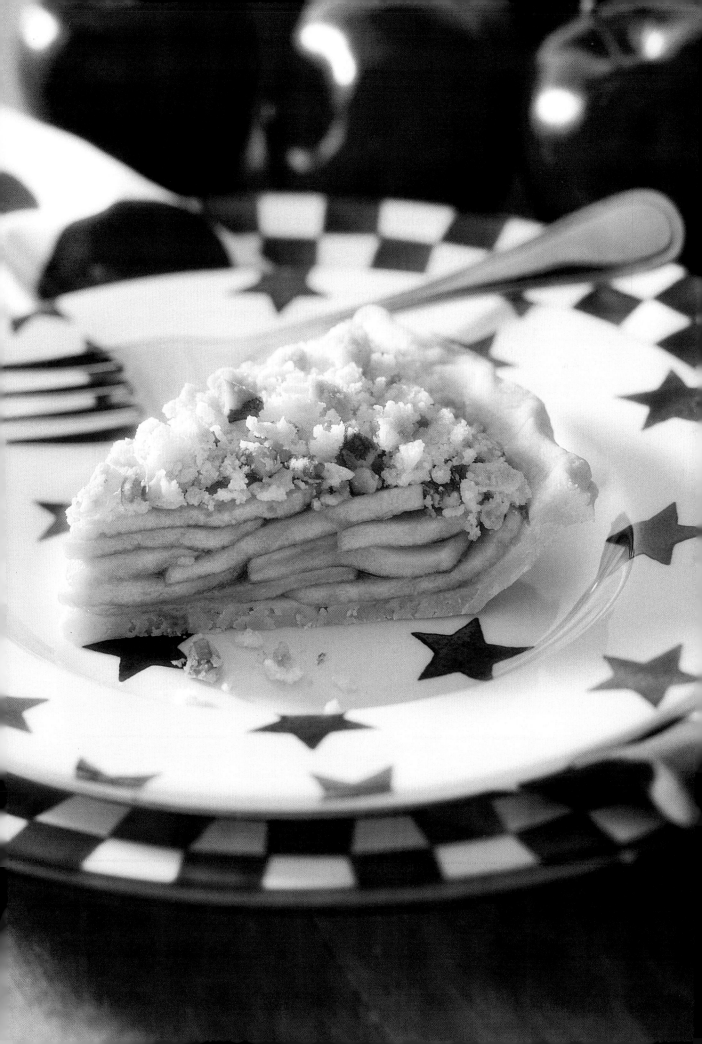

## Rustic Cranberry-Pear Galette

¼ cup granulated sugar, divided
1 tablespoon plus 1 teaspoon cornstarch
2 teaspoons ground cinnamon or apple pie spice
4 cups peeled, thinly sliced Bartlett pears
¼ cup dried cranberries
1 teaspoon vanilla
¼ teaspoon almond extract (optional)
1 refrigerated pie crust, at room temperature
1 egg white
1 tablespoon water

**1.** Preheat oven to 450°F. Coat pizza pan or baking sheet with nonstick cooking spray; set aside.

**2.** Combine all but 1 teaspoon sugar, cornstarch and cinnamon in medium bowl; blend well. Add pears, cranberries, vanilla and almond extract; toss to coat.

**3.** Remove crust from pouch; unfold crust and remove plastic sheets. Place on prepared pan. Spoon pear mixture in center of crust to within 2 inches from edge. Fold edge of crust 2 inches over pear mixture; crimp slightly.

**4.** Combine egg white and water in small bowl; whisk until well blended. Brush outer edges of pie crust with egg white mixture; sprinkle with remaining 1 teaspoon sugar.

**5.** Bake 25 minutes or until pears are tender and crust is golden brown. If edges brown too quickly, cover with foil after 15 minutes of baking. Cool on wire rack 30 minutes. *Makes 8 servings*

### Nutrients per Serving

| | | | | | |
|---|---|---|---|---|---|
| Calories | 227 | Saturated Fat | 3 g | Cholesterol | 5 mg |
| Calories from Fat | 28 % | Protein | 1 g | Sodium | 147 mg |
| Total Fat | 7 g | Carbohydrate | 41 g | Dietary Fiber | 4 g |

DIETARY EXCHANGES: 2 Starch, ½ Fruit, 1 Fat

*Rustic Cranberry-Pear Galette*

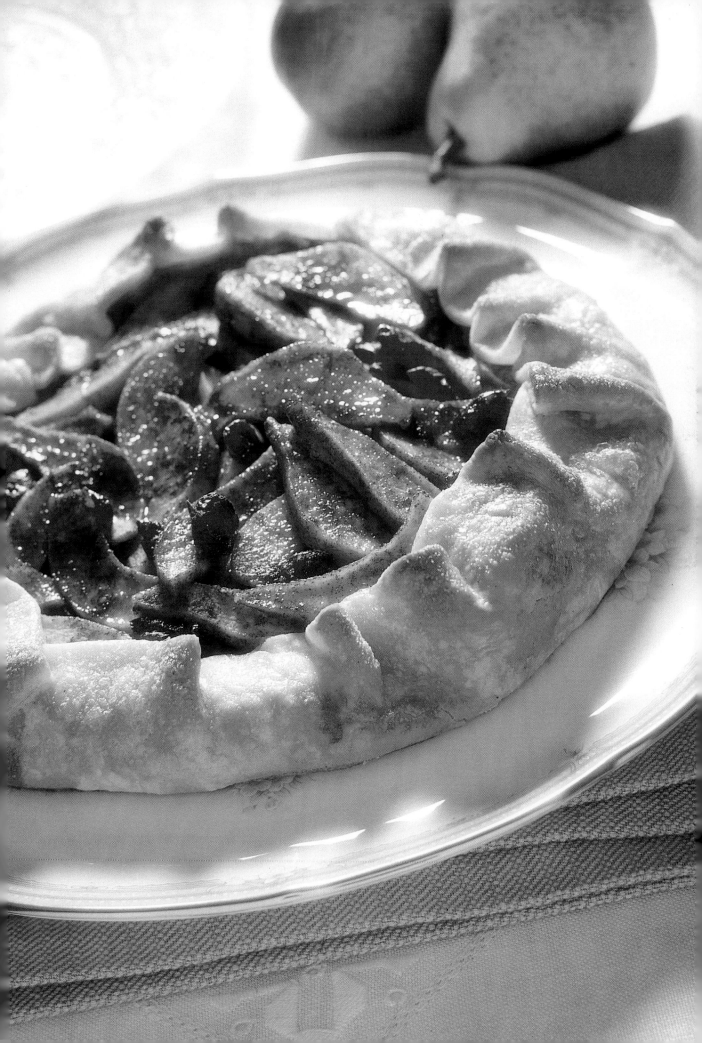

## Apple Crisp

**5 cups thinly sliced Granny Smith apples**
**1 cup apple cider**
**½ cup fat-free butterscotch ice cream topping, divided**
**¼ cup all-purpose flour**
**1 teaspoon ground cinnamon**
**3 cups low-fat granola with raisins**
**3 tablespoons margarine or butter, melted**
   **Low-fat, no-sugar-added ice cream (optional)**

**1.** Preheat oven to 350°F. Lightly coat 8-inch square baking pan with nonstick cooking spray; set aside.

**2.** Combine apples, cider, ¼ cup butterscotch topping, flour and cinnamon in large bowl. Place in prepared pan.

**3.** Combine remaining ¼ cup butterscotch topping, granola and margarine. Dollop over apples.

**4.** Bake, covered, 40 to 45 minutes. Remove cover and bake an additional 15 to 20 minutes or until mixture is bubbly and apples are tender. Serve warm with ice cream, if desired.          *Makes 9 servings*

### Nutrients per Serving

| | | | | | |
|---|---|---|---|---|---|
| Calories | 254 | Saturated Fat | 1 g | Cholesterol | <1 mg |
| Calories from Fat | 21 % | Protein | 3 g | Sodium | 177 mg |
| Total Fat | 6 g | Carbohydrate | 51 g | Dietary Fiber | 4 g |

DIETARY EXCHANGES: 2 Starch, 1 Fruit, 1 Fat

## Eggnog Banana Pie

**32 reduced-fat vanilla wafers**
**3 bananas, divided**
**¼ plus ⅛ teaspoon ground nutmeg, divided**
**2 cups fat-free (skim) milk**
**1 package (8 ounces) reduced-fat cream cheese**
**1 package (4 serving size) sugar-free instant vanilla pudding and pie filling**
**½ teaspoon brandy extract**
**1 cup thawed frozen fat-free nondairy whipped topping**

**1.** Line bottom and side of 9-inch pie pan with vanilla wafers. Slice 2 bananas and arrange evenly on top of wafers. Sprinkle with ¼ teaspoon nutmeg; set aside.

**2.** Place milk, cream cheese, pudding mix and brandy extract in food processor or blender; process until smooth. Stir in whipped topping. Spoon mixture evenly over bananas; sprinkle with remaining ⅛ teaspoon nutmeg. Cover with plastic wrap and refrigerate until ready to serve (no longer than 4 hours). Just before serving, slice remaining banana and arrange decoratively on top of pie.      *Makes 8 servings*

### Nutrients per Serving

| Calories | 214 | Saturated Fat | 4 g | Cholesterol | 14 mg |
| Calories from Fat | 29 % | Protein | 6 g | Sodium | 297 mg |
| Total Fat | 7 g | Carbohydrate | 33 g | Dietary Fiber | 1 g |

DIETARY EXCHANGES: 2 Starch, 1½ Fat

*To add a splash of splendor to this fabulous pie, garnish with edible pansies. These wonderful flowers bring fantastic color to this dessert. Be sure to buy the flowers from a specialty produce market or supermarket that carries gourmet produce. Never buy the flowers from a florist as they could be sprayed with pesticide and should never be eaten.*

## Peach Cobbler

**FILLING**

 6 cups sliced ripe peaches (about 6 medium)
 1 tablespoon fresh lemon or orange juice
 1 tablespoon all-purpose flour
 2 tablespoons sugar
 1 teaspoon ground cinnamon

**TOPPING**

 1½ cups all-purpose flour
 ¼ cup plus 2 teaspoons sugar, divided
 1½ teaspoons baking powder
 ½ cup fat-free (skim) milk
 1 egg
 2 tablespoons margarine or butter, melted
 ½ teaspoon ground cinnamon
  No-sugar-added ice cream (optional)

**1.** Preheat oven to 350°F. Coat 9-inch pie pan with nonstick cooking spray; set aside.

**2.** For filling, mix all filling ingredients in medium bowl; spread into prepared pan.

**3.** For topping, combine 1½ cups flour, ¼ cup sugar and baking powder in medium bowl. Combine milk, egg and margarine in small bowl. Add to flour mixture; stir just until flour is blended. Drop batter by tablespoons on top peach filling. Combine 2 teaspoons sugar and ½ teaspoon cinnamon in small bowl; sprinkle on top.

**4.** Bake 45 to 50 minutes or until toothpick inserted in center comes out clean. Serve warm with ice cream, if desired.     *Makes 9 servings*

### Nutrients per Serving

| | | | | | |
|---|---|---|---|---|---|
| Calories | 201 | Saturated Fat | 1 g | Cholesterol | 24 mg |
| Calories from Fat | 15 % | Protein | 4 g | Sodium | 126 mg |
| Total Fat | 3 g | Carbohydrate | 40 g | Dietary Fiber | 3 g |

DIETARY EXCHANGES: 1½ Starch, 1 Fruit, ½ Fat

*Peach Cobbler*

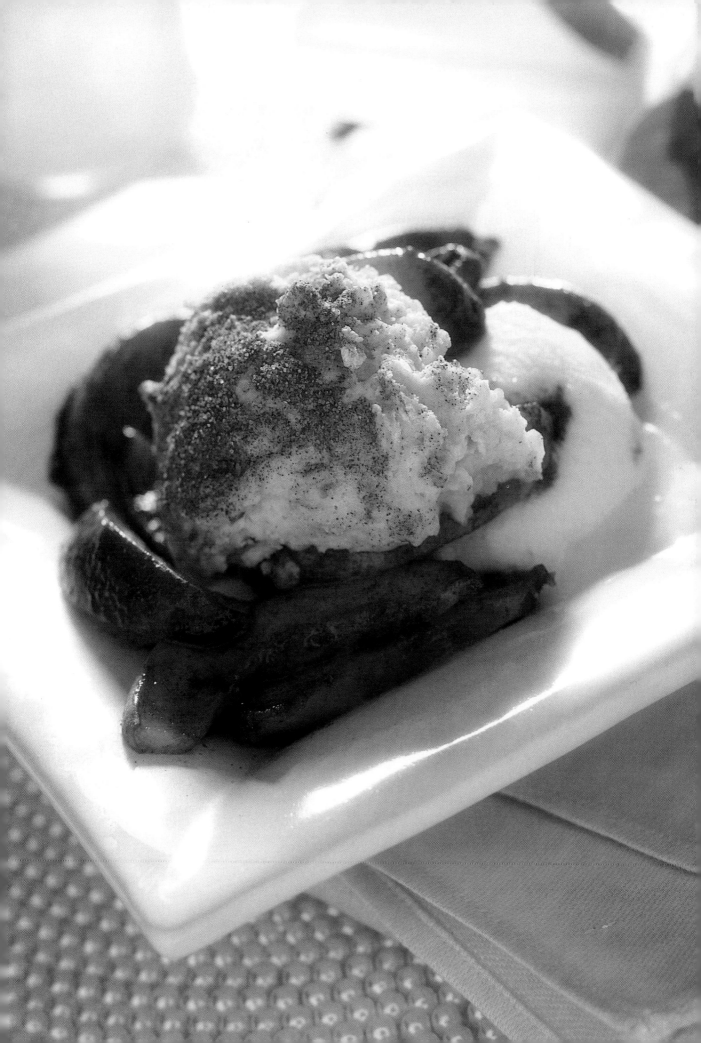

## Farmhouse Lemon Meringue Pie

**1 frozen reduced-fat pie crust**
**4 large eggs, at room temperature**
**3 tablespoons lemon juice**
**2 tablespoons reduced-fat margarine**
**2 teaspoons lemon peel**
**3 drops yellow food coloring (optional)**
**1 cup cold water**
**⅔ cup sugar, divided**
**¼ cup cornstarch**
**⅛ teaspoon salt**
**¼ teaspoon vanilla**

**1.** Preheat oven 425°F. Bake pie crust according to package directions.

**2.** Separate eggs, discarding 2 egg yolks; set aside. Mix lemon juice, margarine, lemon peel and food coloring in small bowl; set aside.

**3.** Combine water, all but 2 tablespoons sugar, cornstarch and salt in medium saucepan; whisk until smooth. Heat over medium-high heat, whisking until mixture begins to boil. Reduce heat to medium. Boil 1 minute, stirring constantly; remove from heat. Stir ¼ cup sugar mixture into egg yolks; whisk until blended. Slowly whisk egg yolk mixture back into sugar mixture. Cook over medium heat 3 minutes, whisking constantly. Remove from heat; stir in lemon juice mixture until blended. Pour into baked pie crust.

**4.** Beat egg whites in large bowl with electric mixer at high speed until soft peaks form. Gradually beat in remaining 2 tablespoons sugar and vanilla; beat until stiff peaks form. Spread meringue over pie filling with rubber spatula, making sure it completely covers filling and touches edge of pie crust. Bake 15 minutes. Remove from oven; cool completely on wire rack. Cover with plastic wrap; refrigerate 8 hours or overnight until setting is firm. *Makes 8 servings*

### Nutrients per Serving

| | | | | | |
|---|---|---|---|---|---|
| Calories | 231 | Saturated Fat | 2 g | Cholesterol | 106 mg |
| Calories from Fat | 34 % | Protein | 4 g | Sodium | 197 mg |
| Total Fat | 9 g | Carbohydrate | 34 g | Dietary Fiber | <1 g |

DIETARY EXCHANGES: 2½ Starch, 1½ Fat

*Farmhouse Lemon Meringue Pie*

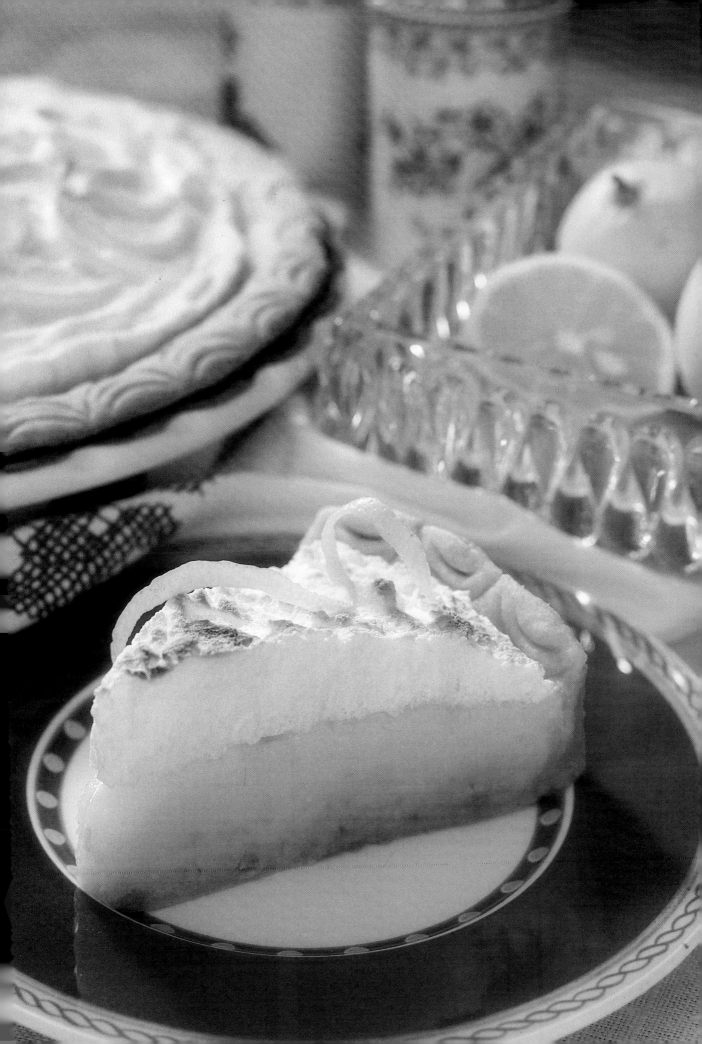

## *Mixed Berry Tart with Ginger-Raspberry Glaze*

**1 refrigerated pie crust, at room temperature**
**¾ cup no-sugar-added seedless raspberry fruit spread**
**½ teaspoon grated fresh ginger *or* ¼ teaspoon ground ginger**
**2 cups fresh or frozen blueberries**
**2 cups fresh or frozen blackberries**
**1 peach, peeled and thinly sliced**

**1.** Preheat oven 450°F. Coat 9-inch pie pan or tart pan with nonstick cooking spray. Carefully place pie crust on bottom of pan. Turn edges of pie crust inward to form ½-inch thick edge. Press edges firmly against sides of pan. Using fork, pierce several times over entire bottom of pan to prevent crust from puffing up while baking. Bake 12 minutes or until golden brown. Cool completely on wire rack.

**2.** Heat fruit spread in small saucepan over high heat; stir until completely melted. Immediately remove from heat; stir in ginger and set aside to cool slightly.

**3.** Combine blueberries, blackberries and all but 2 tablespoons fruit spread mixture; set aside.

**4.** Brush remaining 2 tablespoons fruit spread mixture evenly over bottom of cooled crust. Decoratively arrange peaches on top of crust and mound berries on top of peaches. Refrigerate at least 2 hours.

*Makes 8 servings*

---

### *Nutrients per Serving*

| | | | | | |
|---|---|---|---|---|---|
| Calories | 191 | Saturated Fat | 3 g | Cholesterol | 5 mg |
| Calories from Fat | 33 % | Protein | 1 g | Sodium | 172 mg |
| Total Fat | 7 g | Carbohydrate | 32 g | Dietary Fiber | 3 g |

DIETARY EXCHANGES: 1 Starch, 1 Fruit, 1½ Fat

*Mixed Berry Tart with Ginger-Raspberry Glaze*

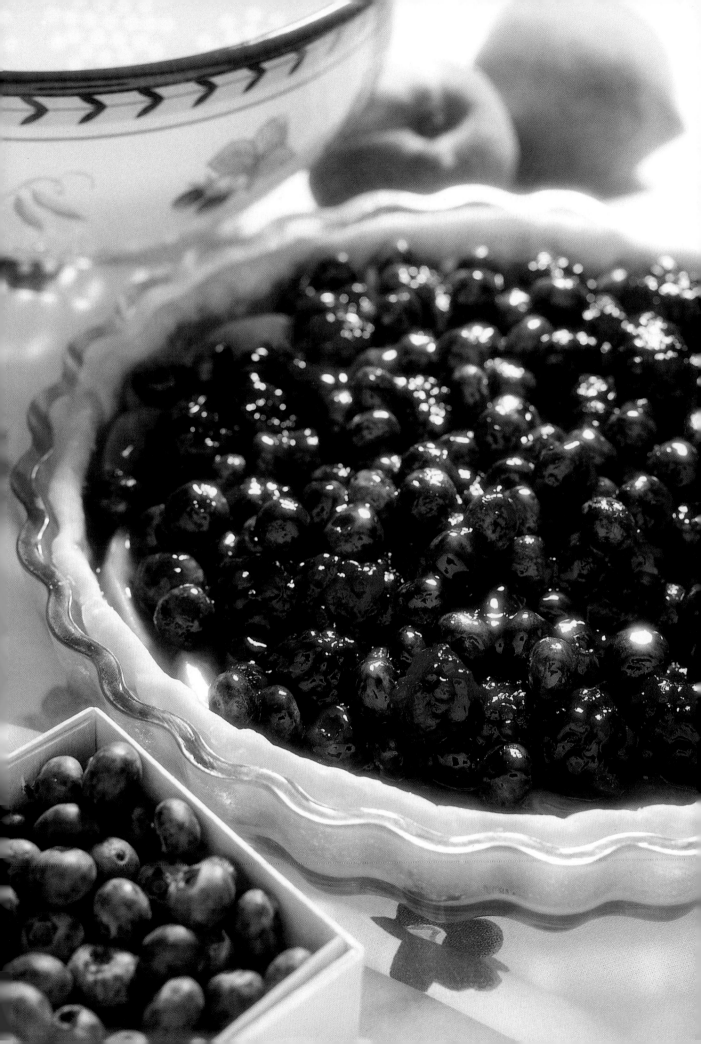

## Mocha Cappuccino Ice Cream Pie

¼ **cup cold water**
1 **tablespoon instant coffee granules**
4 **packets sugar substitute** *or* **equivalent of 8 teaspoons sugar**
½ **teaspoon vanilla**
4 **cups frozen fat-free, no-sugar-added fudge marble ice cream**
1 **vanilla wafer pie crust**

**1.** Combine water, coffee granules, sugar substitute and vanilla in small bowl; stir until granules dissolve. Set aside.

**2.** Combine ice cream and coffee mixture in large bowl; stir gently until liquid is blended into ice cream. Spoon into pie crust; smooth top with rubber spatula.

**3.** Cover with plastic wrap; freeze about 4 hours or until firm.

*Makes 8 servings*

**Variation:** Omit pie crust and serve in dessert cups with biscotti.

### Nutrients per Serving

| | | | | | |
|---|---|---|---|---|---|
| Calories | 201 | Saturated Fat | 2 g | Cholesterol | 9 mg |
| Calories from Fat | 34 % | Protein | 5 g | Sodium | 159 mg |
| Total Fat | 8 g | Carbohydrate | 29 g | Dietary Fiber | 0 g |

DIETARY EXCHANGES: 2 Starch, 1½ Fat

## Blueberry Granola Crumble Pie

**1 package (16 ounces) frozen unsweetened blueberries**
**¼ cup sugar**
**2 tablespoons lemon juice**
**1½ tablespoons cornstarch**
**2 teaspoons vanilla**
**1 frozen reduced-fat pie crust**
**1 cup low-fat granola**

**1.** Preheat oven 425°F. Place baking sheet in oven while preheating.

**2.** Toss blueberries, sugar, lemon juice, cornstarch and vanilla to coat. Spoon blueberry mixture into pie crust; place on heated baking sheet.

**3.** Bake 20 minutes; sprinkle granola evenly over pie. Bake an additional 20 minutes or until pie is bubbly.            *Makes 8 servings*

**Cook's Tip:** If pie is allowed to stand 4 hours or overnight the flavors will blend making a sweeter tasting dessert. This is true with most fruit pies, especially blueberry, cherry and peach pies.

### Nutrients per Serving

| | | | | | |
|---|---|---|---|---|---|
| Calories | 216 | Saturated Fat | 1 g | Cholesterol | 0 mg |
| Calories from Fat | 24 % | Protein | 3 g | Sodium | 126 mg |
| Total Fat | 6 g | Carbohydrate | 39 g | Dietary Fiber | 3 g |

DIETARY EXCHANGES: 2 Starch, ½ Fruit, 1 Fat

# *Company's Coming*

## *Spun Sugar Berries with Yogurt Crème*

**2 cups fresh raspberries***
**1 container (8 ounces) lemon-flavored nonfat yogurt with
    aspartame sweetener**
**1 cup thawed frozen fat-free nondairy whipped topping**
**3 tablespoons sugar**

*\*You may substitute your favorite fresh berry for the fresh raspberries.*

**1.** Arrange berries in 4 glass dessert dishes.

**2.** Combine yogurt and whipped topping in medium bowl. (If not using immediately, cover and refrigerate.) Top berries with yogurt mixture.

**3.** To prepare spun sugar, pour sugar into heavy medium saucepan. Cook over medium-high heat until sugar melts, shaking pan occasionally. *Do not stir.* As sugar begins to melt, reduce heat to low and cook about 10 minutes or until sugar is completely melted and has turned light golden brown.

**4.** Remove from heat; let stand for 1 minute. Coat metal fork with sugar mixture. Drizzle sugar over berries with circular or back and forth motion. Ropes of spun sugar will harden quickly. Garnish as desired. Serve immediately. *Makes 4 servings*

### *Nutrients per Serving*

| | | | | | | | |
|---|---|---|---|---|---|---|---|
| Calories | 119 | Saturated Fat | <1 g | Cholesterol | 0 mg |
| Calories from Fat | 2 % | Protein | 3 g | Sodium | 45 mg |
| Total Fat | <1 g | Carbohydrate | 26 g | Dietary Fiber | 4 g |

DIETARY EXCHANGES: 2 Fruit

*Spun Sugar Berries with Yogurt Crème*

# Company's Coming

## Spun Sugar Berries with Yogurt Crème

**2 cups fresh raspberries***
**1 container (8 ounces) lemon-flavored nonfat yogurt with aspartame sweetener**
**1 cup thawed frozen fat-free nondairy whipped topping**
**3 tablespoons sugar**

*You may substitute your favorite fresh berry for the fresh raspberries.*

**1.** Arrange berries in 4 glass dessert dishes.

**2.** Combine yogurt and whipped topping in medium bowl. (If not using immediately, cover and refrigerate.) Top berries with yogurt mixture.

**3.** To prepare spun sugar, pour sugar into heavy medium saucepan. Cook over medium-high heat until sugar melts, shaking pan occasionally. *Do not stir.* As sugar begins to melt, reduce heat to low and cook about 10 minutes or until sugar is completely melted and has turned light golden brown.

**4.** Remove from heat; let stand for 1 minute. Coat metal fork with sugar mixture. Drizzle sugar over berries with circular or back and forth motion. Ropes of spun sugar will harden quickly. Garnish as desired. Serve immediately.

*Makes 4 servings*

### Nutrients per Serving

| | | | | | | |
|---|---|---|---|---|---|---|
| Calories | 119 | Saturated Fat | <1 g | Cholesterol | 0 mg |
| Calories from Fat | 2% | Protein | 3 g | Sodium | 45 mg |
| Total Fat | <1 g | Carbohydrate | 26 g | Dietary Fiber | 4 g |

DIETARY EXCHANGES: 2 Fruit

*Spun Sugar Berries with Yogurt Crème*

## Blueberry Granola Crumble Pie

**1 package (16 ounces) frozen unsweetened blueberries**
**¼ cup sugar**
**2 tablespoons lemon juice**
**1½ tablespoons cornstarch**
**2 teaspoons vanilla**
**1 frozen reduced-fat pie crust**
**1 cup low-fat granola**

**1.** Preheat oven 425°F. Place baking sheet in oven while preheating.

**2.** Toss blueberries, sugar, lemon juice, cornstarch and vanilla to coat. Spoon blueberry mixture into pie crust; place on heated baking sheet.

**3.** Bake 20 minutes; sprinkle granola evenly over pie. Bake an additional 20 minutes or until pie is bubbly.          *Makes 8 servings*

**Cook's Tip:** If pie is allowed to stand 4 hours or overnight the flavors will blend making a sweeter tasting dessert. This is true with most fruit pies, especially blueberry, cherry and peach pies.

### Nutrients per Serving

| | | | | | | |
|---|---|---|---|---|---|---|
| Calories | 216 | Saturated Fat | 1 g | Cholesterol | 0 mg |
| Calories from Fat | 24% | Protein | 3 g | Sodium | 126 mg |
| Total Fat | 6 g | Carbohydrate | 39 g | Dietary Fiber | 3 g |

DIETARY EXCHANGES: 2 Starch, ½ Fruit, 1 Fat

## Caffè en Forchetta

2 cups reduced-fat (2%) milk
1 cup cholesterol-free egg substitute
½ cup sugar
2 tablespoons no-sugar-added mocha-flavored instant coffee
   Grated chocolate or 6 chocolate-covered coffee beans
   (optional)

1. Preheat oven to 325°F.

2. Combine all ingredients in medium bowl except grated chocolate. Whisk until instant coffee has dissolved and mixture is foamy. Pour into six individual custard cups. Place cups in 13×9-inch baking pan. Fill with hot water halfway up side of cups.

3. Bake 55 to 60 minutes or until knife inserted halfway between center and edge comes out clean. Serve warm or at room temperature. Garnish with grated chocolate or chocolate-covered coffee bean , if desired.

*Makes 6 servings*

### Nutrients per Serving

| | | | | | |
|---|---|---|---|---|---|
| Calories | 111 | Saturated Fat | 1 g | Cholesterol | 6 mg |
| Calories from Fat | 16 % | Protein | 7 g | Sodium | 136 mg |
| Total Fat | 2 g | Carbohydrate | 17 g | Dietary Fiber | 0 g |

DIETARY EXCHANGES: 1 Starch, 1 Lean Meat

*Enjoy your after dinner coffee a whole new way. Translated from Italian, Caffè en Forchetta literally means "coffee on a fork." However, a spoon is recommended when serving this wonderfully creamy dessert.*

*Caffè en Forchetta*

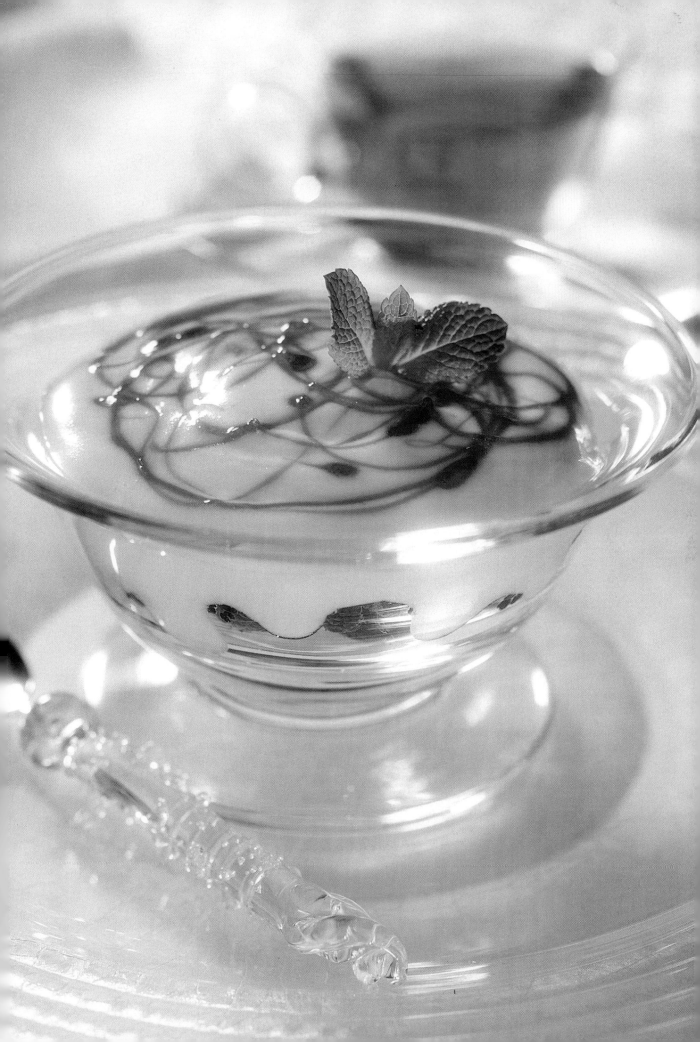

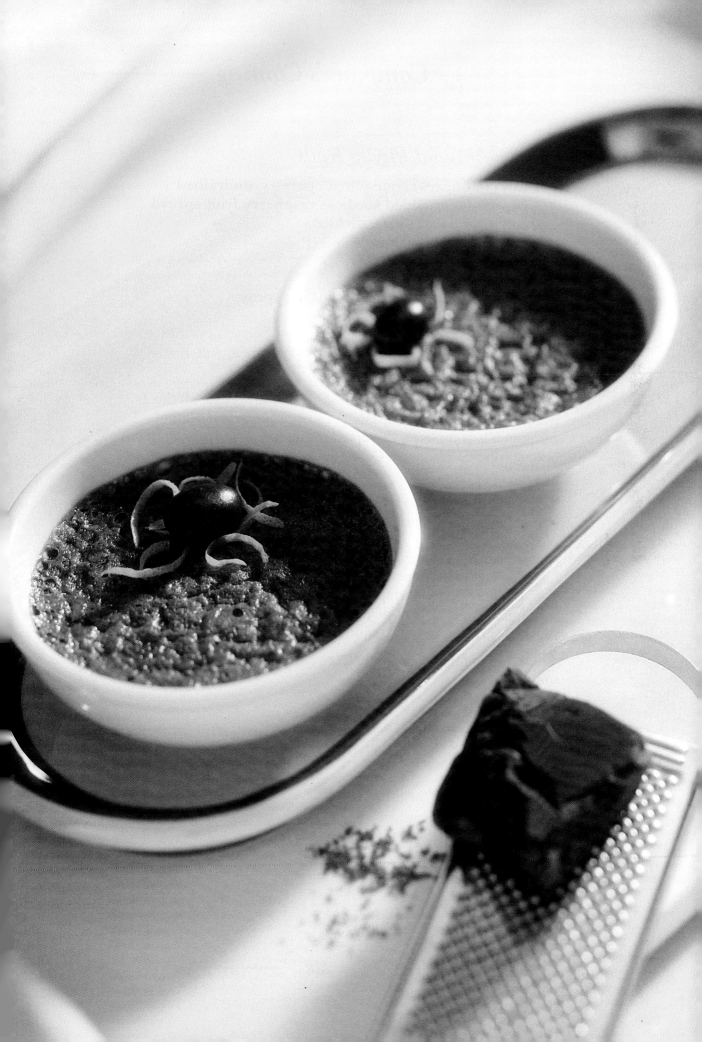

## Cherry-Almond Phyllo Rolls

**1 can (16 ounces) sour pitted cherries, undrained**
**⅓ cup no-sugar-added seedless raspberry fruit spread**
**⅓ cup granulated sugar, divided**
**2 tablespoons cornstarch**
**½ teaspoon almond extract**
**16 sheets phyllo dough**
**Butter-flavored nonstick cooking spray**
**½ cup sliced almonds**

**1.** Preheat oven 400°F. Coat nonstick baking sheet with nonstick cooking spray; set aside.

**2.** Combine cherries with juice, raspberry fruit spread, all but 1 tablespoon sugar and cornstarch in small saucepan. Stir until cornstarch is completely dissolved. Bring to a boil over medium-high heat, stirring occasionally. Continue boiling and gently stirring one minute. Remove from heat and stir in almond extract; set aside.

**3.** Place 2 sheets phyllo dough on work surface. Keep remaining sheets covered with plastic wrap and damp kitchen towel. Spray top sheet of phyllo dough with nonstick cooking spray; fold in half crosswise and spray again. Spoon ⅓ cup cherry mixture to within 3 inches of bottom long edge. Fold up bottom edge. Fold in both sides. Beginning at long side, roll up jelly-roll fashion; place on prepared baking sheet. Repeat with remaining sheets of phyllo and cherry mixture. Sprinkle remaining sugar over rolls; top with almonds.

**4.** Bake 20 minutes; remove from oven and let stand 15 minutes before serving.

*Makes 8 servings*

### *Nutrients per Serving*

| | | | | | |
|---|---|---|---|---|---|
| Calories | 247 | Saturated Fat | 1 g | Cholesterol | 0 mg |
| Calories from Fat | 22 % | Protein | 4 g | Sodium | 201 mg |
| Total Fat | 6 g | Carbohydrate | 40 g | Dietary Fiber | 2 g |

DIETARY EXCHANGES: 2 Starch, 1 Fruit, 1 Fat

## Baked Orange Custard with Strawberries

¾ **cup cholesterol-free egg substitute**
½ **cup sugar**
1 **can (12 ounces) nonfat evaporated milk**
¼ **cup heavy cream**
2 **tablespoons fresh squeezed orange juice**
1 **tablespoon grated orange peel**
1 **teaspoon vanilla**
2½ **cups fresh sliced strawberries**
3 **packets sugar substitute *or* equivalent of 2 tablespoons sugar**

**1.** Preheat oven to 350°F. Combine egg substitute, sugar, evaporated milk, cream, orange juice, orange peel and vanilla in medium bowl until well blended. Pour mixture into 6 (6-ounce) custard cups or ramekins. Place custard cups in 13×9-inch baking pan. Fill with hot water halfway up side of cups. Bake 30 to 35 minutes or until knife inserted halfway between center and edge comes out clean.

**2.** Remove from oven; let cups remain in hot water bath until they reach room temperature.

**3.** While custards cool, gently toss sliced strawberries with sugar substitute; set aside.

**4.** Serve custards at room temperature or cold. Top with strawberries.

*Makes 6 servings*

### Nutrients per Serving

| | | | | | |
|---|---|---|---|---|---|
| Calories | 190 | Saturated Fat | 2 g | Cholesterol | 16 mg |
| Calories from Fat | 18% | Protein | 9 g | Sodium | 128 mg |
| Total Fat | 4 g | Carbohydrate | 30 g | Dietary Fiber | 2 g |

DIETARY EXCHANGES: 2 Starch, ½ Lean Meat

## Tropical Fruit Coconut Tart

**1 cup cornflakes, crushed**
**1 can (3½ ounces) sweetened flaked coconut**
**2 egg whites**
**1 can (15¼ ounces) pineapple tidbits in juice**
**2 teaspoons cornstarch**
**2 packets sugar substitute** *or* **equivalent of 4 teaspoons sugar**
**1 teaspoon coconut extract (optional)**
**1 mango, peeled and thinly sliced**
**1 banana, thinly sliced**

**1.** Preheat oven to 425°F. Coat 9-inch springform pan with nonstick cooking spray; set aside.

**2.** Combine cereal, coconut and egg whites in medium bowl; toss gently to blend. Place coconut mixture in prepared pan; press firmly to coat bottom and ½ inch up side of pan.

**3.** Bake 8 minutes or until edge begins to brown. Cool completely on wire rack.

**4.** Drain pineapple, reserving pineapple juice. Combine pineapple juice and cornstarch in small saucepan; stir until cornstarch is dissolved. Bring to a boil over high heat. Continue boiling 1 minute, stirring constantly. Remove from heat; cool completely. Stir in sugar substitute and coconut extract. Combine pineapple, mango slices and banana slices in medium bowl. Spoon into pan; drizzle with pineapple sauce. Cover with plastic wrap and refrigerate 2 hours. Garnish with pineapple leaves, if desired. *Makes 8 servings*

**Note:** The crust may be made 24 hours in advance, if desired.

### Nutrients per Serving

| | | | | | |
|---|---|---|---|---|---|
| Calories | 139 | Saturated Fat | 4 g | Cholesterol | 0 mg |
| Calories from Fat | 25 % | Protein | 2 g | Sodium | 59 mg |
| Total Fat | 4 g | Carbohydrate | 25 g | Dietary Fiber | 2 g |

DIETARY EXCHANGES: 1 Starch, ½ Fruit, 1 Fat

*Tropical Fruit Coconut Tart*

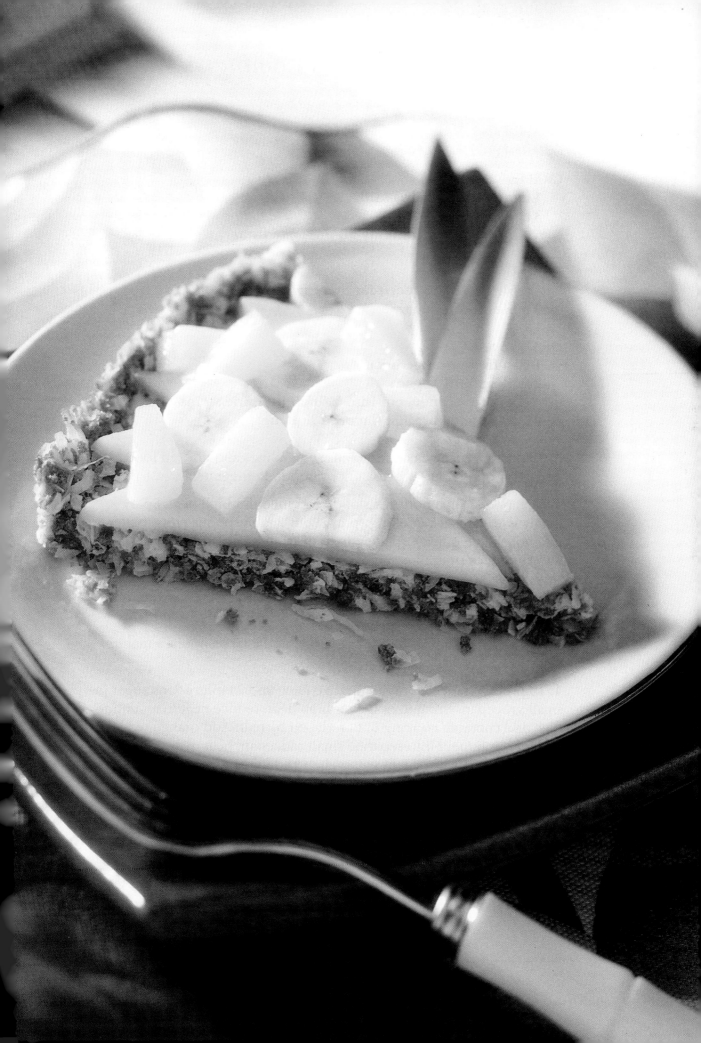

## *Sinfully Slim Crêpes Suzette*

**CRÊPES**
> 1 cup fat-free (skim) milk
> 3 egg whites
> ¼ cup plus 2 tablespoons all-purpose flour

**FILLING**
> 2½ tablespoons reduced-fat margarine
> 2 tablespoons sugar

**ORANGE SAUCE**
> 1 cup fresh orange juice
> 2 tablespoons sugar
> Peel of 1 orange, cut into ⅛-inch julienne strips
> 2 tablespoons orange-flavored liqueur

**1.** To prepare crêpes, combine milk, egg whites and flour in food processor or blender; process until smooth. Refrigerate at least 1 hour.

**2.** Heat 6- or 7-inch nonstick skillet over medium-high heat. Spray lightly with nonstick cooking spray. Pour 2 tablespoons crêpe batter into hot skillet; quickly rotate pan to distribute batter evenly. Cook 1 to 2 minutes or until nicely browned. Flip crêpe and cook on other side about 30 seconds. Stack crêpes on clean kitchen towel. Repeat with remaining batter, spraying skillet with nonstick cooking spray before each crêpe.

**3.** To prepare filling, combine margarine and 2 tablespoons sugar in small bowl; set aside.

**4.** To prepare sauce, combine orange juice and 2 tablespoons sugar in small saucepan. Bring to boil over high heat; reduce heat to medium-high and continue cooking until reduced by half. Add orange peel; set aside. Pour liqueur into separate small saucepan; heat over medium-high heat until warm. Light with match and immediately stop flame with lid. Combine liqueur and orange sauce; keep warm. Set aside.

**5.** To serve, spread each crêpe with about ½ teaspoon filling mixture. Fold crêpes in half, then in half again to form a triangle. Arrange 2 crêpes on each dessert plate; repeat with remaining crêpes. Top each serving with about 1 tablespoon orange sauce; serve warm.

*Makes 6 servings (12 to 14 crêpes)*

### Nutrients per Serving

| | | | | | |
|---|---|---|---|---|---|
| Calories | 139 | Saturated Fat | <1 g | Cholesterol | 1 mg |
| Calories from Fat | 16 % | Protein | 4 g | Sodium | 106 mg |
| Total Fat | 3 g | Carbohydrate | 23 g | Dietary Fiber | <1 g |

DIETARY EXCHANGES: 1½ Starch, ½ Fat

## Fruited Trifle

**1¾ cups fat-free (skim) milk**
**1 package (4 serving size) instant sugar-free vanilla pudding and pie filling**
**4 ounces Neufchâtel cheese, softened**
**12 to 16 whole ladyfingers**
**2 tablespoons cream sherry, divided (optional)**
**2 cups fresh or frozen raspberries**
**½ cup thawed frozen fat-free nondairy whipped topping**

**1.** Whisk together milk and pudding mix in large bowl. Beat in Neufchâtel with electric mixer at medium speed until smooth; set aside.

**2.** Place half the ladyfingers on bottom of 8- to 10-inch glass serving dish. Top with 1 tablespoon sherry. Spread half the pudding mixture over ladyfingers. Arrange raspberries over pudding, reserving a few for garnish. Repeat layers with remaining ingredients.

**3.** Top with whipped topping. Refrigerate 1 hour. Garnish with reserved raspberries just before serving. *Makes 8 servings*

### Nutrients per Serving

| | | | | | |
|---|---|---|---|---|---|
| Calories | 145 | Saturated Fat | 2 g | Cholesterol | 68 mg |
| Calories from Fat | 25 % | Protein | 5 g | Sodium | 122 mg |
| Total Fat | 4 g | Carbohydrate | 21 g | Dietary Fiber | 2 g |

DIETARY EXCHANGES: 1½ Starch, ½ Fat

## Cider-Poached Apples with Cinnamon Yogurt

    **2 cups apple cider or apple juice**
    **1 stick cinnamon *or* ½ teaspoon ground cinnamon**
    **2 Golden Delicious apples, peeled, halved and cored**
    **½ cup vanilla-flavored nonfat yogurt with aspartame**
        **sweetener**
    **½ teaspoon ground cinnamon**
    **½ cup chopped pecans, toasted**

**1.** Bring apple cider and cinnamon stick to a boil in 2- to 3-quart sauce pan over high heat. Let boil, uncovered, about 25 minutes or until liquid is reduced to about 1 cup.

**2.** Add apples; cover and simmer about 10 minutes or until apples are just tender. Gently remove apple halves and poaching liquid from saucepan. Refrigerate until cooled.

**3.** Combine yogurt and ground cinnamon in small bowl; reserve 2 tablespoons. Divide remaining yogurt mixture evenly among 4 dessert dishes. Place apple halves on top of sauce. Sprinkle each apple half with toasted pecans. Drizzle with reserved yogurt mixture.

*Makes 4 servings*

*Nutrients per Serving*

| | | | | | |
|---|---|---|---|---|---|
| Calories | 159 | Saturated Fat | <1 g | Cholesterol | 0 mg |
| Calories from Fat | 27 % | Protein | 2 g | Sodium | 21 mg |
| Total Fat | 5 g | Carbohydrate | 30 g | Dietary Fiber | 2 g |

DIETARY EXCHANGES: 2 Fruit, 1 Fat

*To toast the pecans, spread in a single layer on a baking sheet and toast in a preheated 350°F oven for 8 to 10 minutes or until very lightly browned. Use them immediately or store them in a covered container in the refrigerator.*

*Cider-Poached Apple with Cinnamon Yogurt*

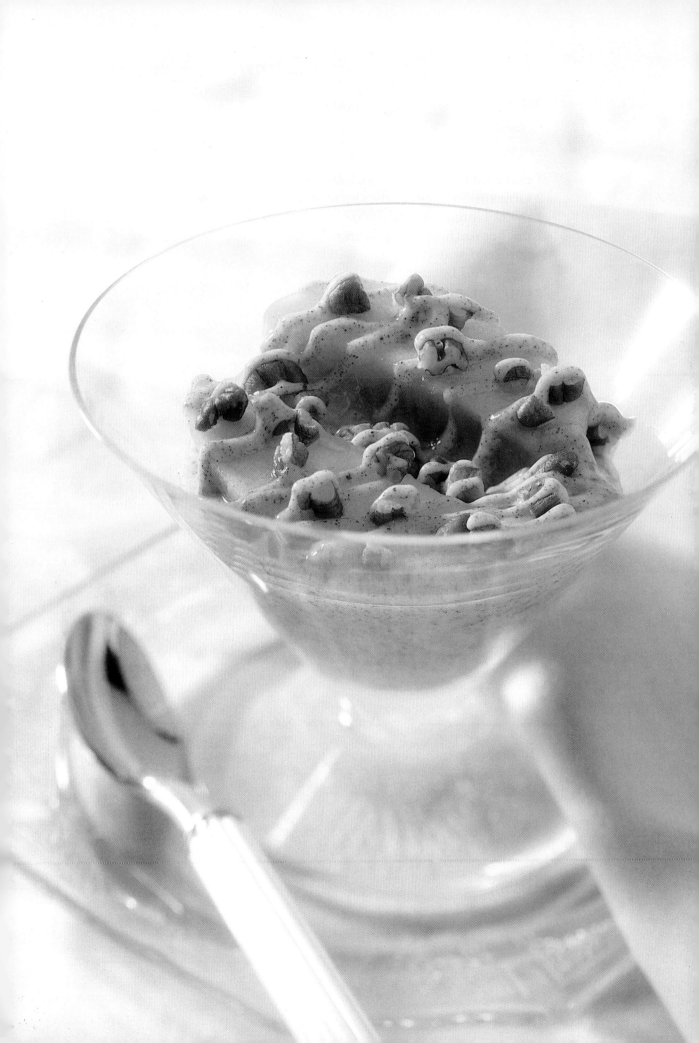

## Lemon Mousse Squares

1 cup graham cracker crumbs
2 tablespoons reduced-calorie margarine, melted
1 packet sugar substitute *or* equivalent of 2 teaspoons sugar
1 packet unflavored gelatin
⅓ cup cold water
2 eggs, well beaten
½ cup lemon juice
¼ cup sugar
2 teaspoon grated lemon peel
2 cups thawed frozen fat-free nondairy whipped topping
1 container (8 ounces) lemon-flavored nonfat yogurt with aspartame sweetener

**1.** Stir together graham cracker crumbs, melted margarine and sugar substitute in 9-inch square baking pan sprayed with nonstick cooking spray. Press into bottom of pan with fork; set aside.

**2.** Combine gelatin and cold water in small microwavable bowl; let stand 2 minutes. Microwave at HIGH 40 seconds to dissolve gelatin; set aside.

**3.** Combine eggs, lemon juice, sugar and lemon peel in top of double boiler. Cook, stirring constantly, over boiling water, about 4 minutes or until thickened. Remove from heat; stir in gelatin. Refrigerate about 25 minutes, or until mixture is thoroughly cooled and begins to set.

**4.** Gently whip together lemon-gelatin mixture, whipped topping and lemon yogurt. Pour into prepared crust. Refrigerate 1 hour or until firm.

*Makes 9 servings*

### Nutrients per Serving

| | | | | | |
|---|---|---|---|---|---|
| Calories | 154 | Saturated Fat | 1 g | Cholesterol | 47 mg |
| Calories from Fat | 29 % | Protein | 3 g | Sodium | 124 mg |
| Total Fat | 5 g | Carbohydrate | 24 g | Dietary Fiber | 1 g |

DIETARY EXCHANGES: 1½ Starch, 1 Fat

*Lemon Mousse Squares*

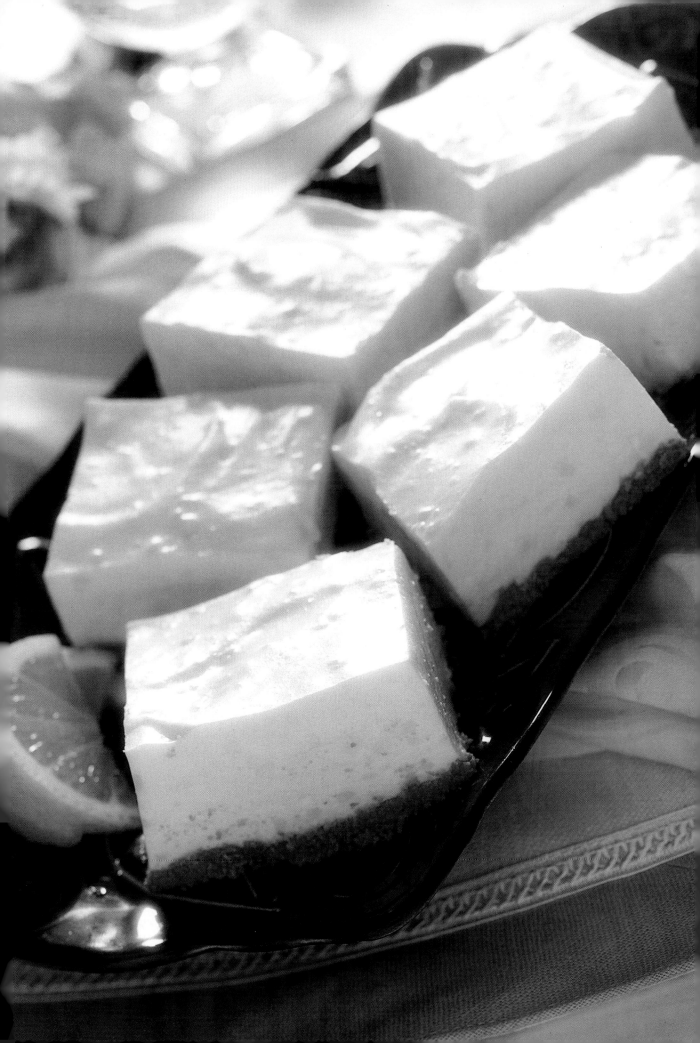

## Strawberry-Peach Cream Puffs

    1 cup water
    ¼ cup margarine
    1 cup all-purpose flour
    4 eggs
    1 quart strawberries, stemmed and quartered
  1½ cups diced peaches or nectarines
    6 packets sugar substitute *or* equivalent of ¼ cup sugar
    1 teaspoon vanilla
    ½ teaspoon almond extract
    2 cups fat-free vanilla ice cream or 2 cups thawed frozen
       fat-free nondairy whipped topping
    1 tablespoon powdered sugar

**1.** Preheat oven to 400°F. Combine water and margarine in medium saucepan. Bring to boil over high heat. Reduce heat to low; stir in flour until well blended. Remove from heat, stir in eggs one at a time until well blended.

**2.** Spoon 4 tablespoons batter side by side to form cloverleaf on ungreased baking sheet. Repeat with remaining batter. Bake 35 minutes or until golden brown.

**3.** Combine strawberries, peaches, sugar substitute, vanilla and almond extract in medium bowl. Place ¾ cup strawberry mixture in food processor or blender; process until smooth. Return to remaining strawberry mixture; set aside.

**4.** Once cream puffs are done, place baking sheet on wire rack; cool completely. Cut each cream puff in half crosswise. Spoon ¼ cup ice cream or whipped topping on bottom half of each cream puff. Spoon about ½ cup strawberry mixture on top of ice cream; top with top half of cream puff. Sprinkle with powdered sugar. Serve immediately.

*Makes 8 servings*

### Nutrients per Serving

| Calories | 235 | Saturated Fat | 2 g | Cholesterol | 106 mg |
|---|---|---|---|---|---|
| Calories from Fat | 34 % | Protein | 8 g | Sodium | 134 mg |
| Total Fat | 9 g | Carbohydrate | 32 g | Dietary Fiber | 3 g |

DIETARY EXCHANGES: 1½ Starch, 1 Fruit, 1½ Fat

*Strawberry-Peach Cream Puff*

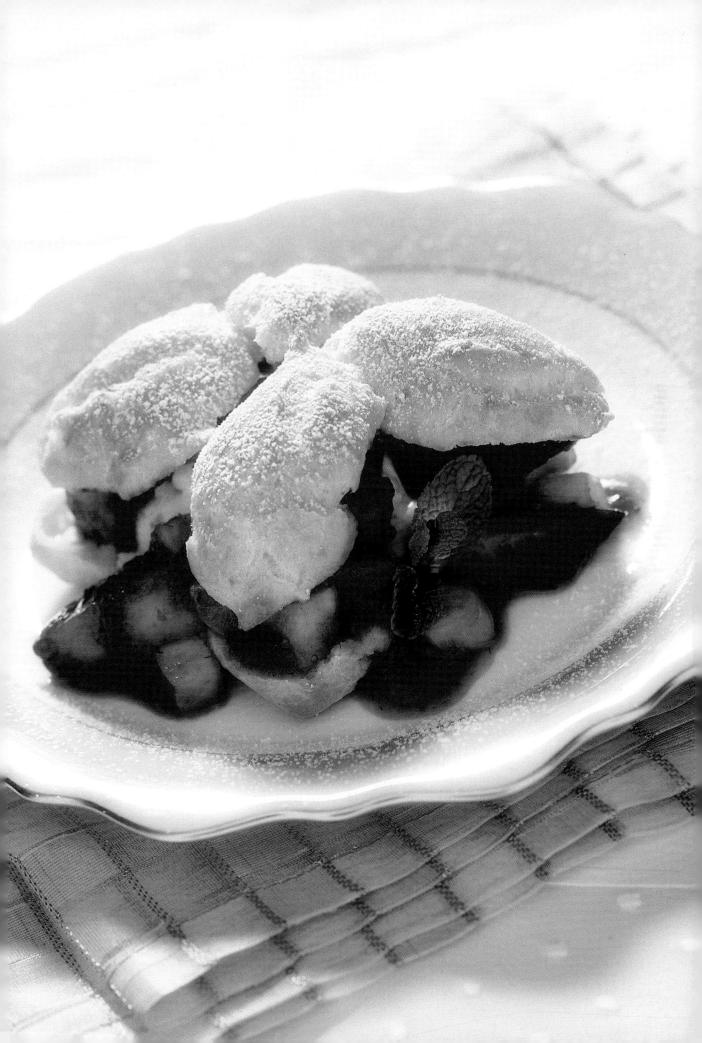

## Layered Fresh Fruit Jewels

**1 cup cake flour**
**⅓ cup sugar**
**1 teaspoon baking powder**
    **Dash salt**
**¼ cup water**
**3 tablespoons canola oil**
**1½ teaspoons vanilla**
**3 egg whites, at room temperature**
**½ teaspoon cream of tartar**
**3 cups assorted fresh fruit, such as strawberries, kiwis,**
    **blueberries, pineapple, raspberries, apricots or plums**
**⅓ cup no-sugar-added apricot spread, strained**
**1 tablespoon orange-flavored liqueur or water**

**1.** Preheat oven to 350°F. Lightly grease 13×9-inch baking pan; set aside.

**2.** Combine flour, sugar, baking powder and salt in large bowl. Add water, oil and vanilla; set aside.

**3.** Beat egg whites in large bowl with electric mixer at high speed until foamy. Add cream of tartar; continue beating at high speed until stiff peaks form.

**4.** Gently fold egg whites into cake batter. Pour into prepared pan; smooth surface of batter. Bake 15 minutes or until toothpick inserted in center comes out clean; cool 5 minutes. Gently turn cake out of pan; cool completely.

**5.** Cut cake lengthwise in half, then cut crosswise into 14 rectangles of equal size.

**6.** Combine spread and liqueur in small microwavable bowl. Microwave at HIGH 20 seconds or until warmed through; set aside.

**7.** To assemble, place 1 cake slice on each dessert plate. Brush warmed glaze on cake; top with single layer of fruit. Repeat layer ending with fruit.

*Makes 7 servings*

### Nutrients per Serving

| | | | | | | |
|---|---|---|---|---|---|---|
| Calories | 214 | Saturated Fat | <1 g | Cholesterol | 0 mg |
| Calories from Fat | 26 % | Protein | 3 g | Sodium | 111 mg |
| Total Fat | 6 g | Carbohydrate | 35 g | Dietary Fiber | 2 g |

DIETARY EXCHANGES: 1½ Starch, 1 Fruit, 1 Fat

# My Favorites

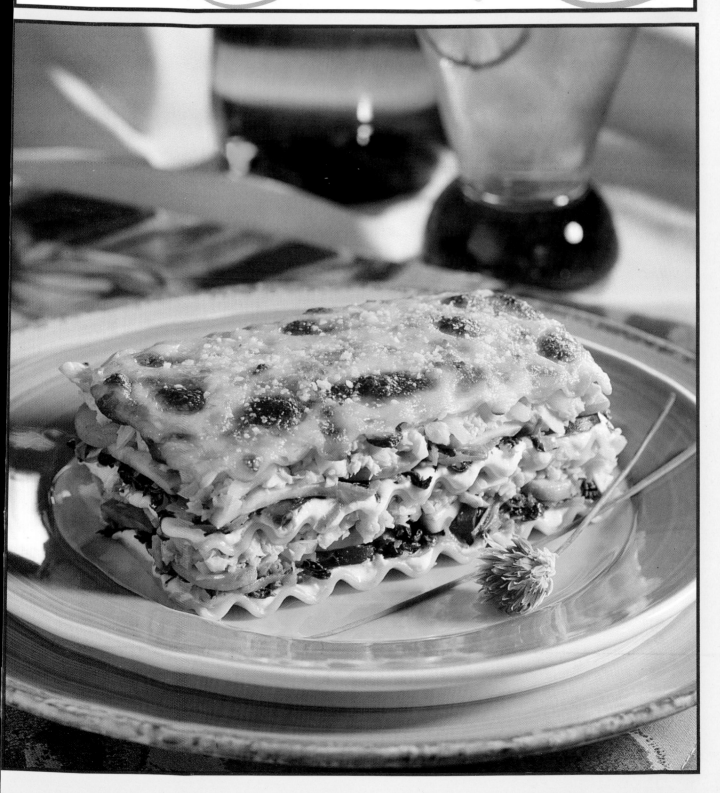

# *My Favorite Recipes*

Favorite recipe: _____

Favorite recipe from: _____

Ingredients: _____

_____

_____

_____

_____

_____

Method: _____

_____

_____

_____

_____

_____

_____

_____

_____

_____

_____

_____

## *My Favorite Recipes*

**Favorite recipe:** _____

**Favorite recipe from:** _____

**Ingredients:** _____

_____

_____

_____

_____

_____

**Method:** _____

_____

_____

_____

_____

_____

_____

_____

_____

_____

_____

# *My Favorite Recipes*

**Favorite recipe:** _____

**Favorite recipe from:** _____

**Ingredients:** _____

_____

_____

_____

_____

_____

**Method:** _____

_____

_____

_____

_____

_____

_____

_____

_____

_____

_____

## My Favorite Recipes

Favorite recipe: _____

Favorite recipe from: _____

Ingredients: _____

_____

_____

_____

_____

_____

Method: _____

_____

_____

_____

_____

_____

_____

_____

_____

_____

_____

# *My Favorite Recipes*

**Favorite recipe:** _____

**Favorite recipe from:** _____

**Ingredients:** _____
_____
_____
_____
_____

**Method:** _____
_____
_____
_____
_____
_____
_____
_____
_____
_____

**Favorite recipe:** _____

**Favorite recipe from:** _____

**Ingredients:** _____

_____

_____

_____

_____

**Method:** _____

_____

_____

_____

_____

_____

_____

_____

_____

_____

_____

# *My Favorite Recipes*

**Favorite recipe:** _____

**Favorite recipe from:** _____

**Ingredients:** _____

_____

_____

_____

_____

_____

**Method:** _____

_____

_____

_____

_____

_____

_____

_____

_____

_____

# *My Favorite Recipes*

Favorite recipe: _____

Favorite recipe from: _____

Ingredients: _____

_____

_____

_____

_____

Method: _____

_____

_____

_____

_____

_____

_____

_____

_____

_____

# *My Favorite Recipes*

**Favorite recipe:** _____

**Favorite recipe from:** _____

**Ingredients:** _____

_____

_____

_____

_____

**Method:** _____

_____

_____

_____

_____

_____

_____

_____

_____

**Favorite recipe:** _____

**Favorite recipe from:** _____

**Ingredients:** _____

_____

_____

_____

_____

**Method:** _____

_____

_____

_____

_____

_____

_____

_____

_____

_____

# *My Favorite Recipes*

Favorite recipe: _____

Favorite recipe from: _____

Ingredients: _____

_____

_____

_____

_____

Method: _____

_____

_____

_____

_____

_____

_____

_____

_____

_____

# *My Favorite Recipes*

**Favorite recipe:** _____

**Favorite recipe from:** _____

**Ingredients:** _____

_____

_____

_____

_____

_____

**Method:** _____

_____

_____

_____

_____

_____

_____

_____

_____

_____

_____

# *My Favorite Recipes*

Favorite recipe: _____

Favorite recipe from: _____

Ingredients: _____

_____

_____

_____

_____

_____

Method: _____

_____

_____

_____

_____

_____

_____

_____

_____

_____

**Favorite recipe:** _____

**Favorite recipe from:** _____

**Ingredients:** _____

_____

_____

_____

_____

_____

**Method:** _____

_____

_____

_____

_____

_____

_____

_____

_____

_____

_____

# My Favorite Recipes

**Favorite recipe:** _____

**Favorite recipe from:** _____

**Ingredients:** _____

_____

_____

_____

_____

_____

**Method:** _____

_____

_____

_____

_____

_____

_____

_____

_____

_____

_____

## *My Favorite Recipes*

**Favorite recipe:** _____

**Favorite recipe from:** _____

**Ingredients:** _____

_____

_____

_____

_____

**Method:** _____

_____

_____

_____

_____

_____

_____

_____

_____

_____

# *My Favorite Recipes*

**Favorite recipe:** _____

**Favorite recipe from:** _____

**Ingredients:** _____

_____

_____

_____

_____

_____

**Method:** _____

_____

_____

_____

_____

_____

_____

_____

_____

_____

_____

# My Favorite Recipes

Favorite recipe: _____

Favorite recipe from: _____

Ingredients: _____

_____

_____

_____

_____

Method: _____

_____

_____

_____

_____

_____

_____

_____

_____

_____

_____

# *My Favorite Recipes*

**Favorite recipe:** _____

**Favorite recipe from:** _____

**Ingredients:** _____

_____

_____

_____

_____

_____

**Method:** _____

_____

_____

_____

_____

_____

_____

_____

_____

_____

_____

# *My Favorite Recipes*

Favorite recipe: _____

Favorite recipe from: _____

Ingredients: _____

_____

_____

_____

_____

_____

Method: _____

_____

_____

_____

_____

_____

_____

_____

_____

_____

_____

_____

## *My Favorite Dinner Party*

**Date:** _____

**Occasion:** _____

_____

**Guests:** _____

_____

_____

_____

_____

**Menu:** _____

_____

_____

_____

_____

_____

_____

_____

_____

_____

_____

_____

# *My Favorite Dinner Party*

**Date:** _____

**Occasion:** _____
_____

**Guests:** _____
_____
_____
_____
_____

**Menu:** _____
_____
_____
_____
_____
_____
_____
_____
_____
_____
_____

# *My Favorite Dinner Party*

**Date:** _____

**Occasion:** _____
_____

**Guests:** _____
_____
_____
_____
_____

**Menu:** _____
_____
_____
_____
_____
_____
_____
_____
_____
_____
_____
_____

# *My Favorite Dinner Party*

**Date:** _____

**Occasion:** _____

_____

**Guests:** _____

_____

_____

_____

_____

**Menu:** _____

_____

_____

_____

_____

_____

_____

_____

_____

_____

_____

_____

# My Favorite Take-Along Treats

**Date:** _____

**Occasion:** _____

_____

**Guests:** _____

_____

_____

_____

_____

**Menu:** _____

_____

_____

_____

_____

_____

_____

_____

_____

_____

_____

# *My Favorite Take-Along Treats*

**Date:** _____

**Occasion:** _____

_____

**Guests:** _____

_____

_____

_____

_____

**Menu:** _____

_____

_____

_____

_____

_____

_____

_____

_____

_____

_____

_____

# *My Favorite Take-Along Treats*

**Date:** _____

**Occasion:** _____

_____

**Guests:** _____

_____

_____

_____

_____

**Menu:** _____

_____

_____

_____

_____

_____

_____

_____

_____

_____

_____

# *My Favorite Take-Along Treats*

**Date:** _____

**Occasion:** _____

_____

**Guests:** _____

_____

_____

_____

_____

**Menu:** _____

_____

_____

_____

_____

_____

_____

_____

_____

_____

_____

_____

## *My Favorite Friends*

**Friend:** _____

**Favorite foods:** _____

_____

_____

_____

_____

_____

**Don't serve:** _____

_____

_____

_____

_____

_____

_____

_____

_____

_____

_____

## My Favorite Friends

**Friend:** _____

**Favorite foods:** _____

_____

_____

_____

_____

_____

**Don't serve:** _____

_____

_____

_____

_____

_____

_____

_____

_____

_____

_____

_____

_____

# My Favorite Friends

**Friend:** _____

**Favorite foods:** _____

_____

_____

_____

_____

_____

**Don't serve:** _____

_____

_____

_____

_____

_____

_____

_____

_____

_____

_____

_____

_____

**Friend:** _____

**Favorite foods:** _____

_____

_____

_____

_____

_____

**Don't serve:** _____

_____

_____

_____

_____

_____

_____

_____

_____

_____

_____

_____

_____

# Hints, Tips & Index

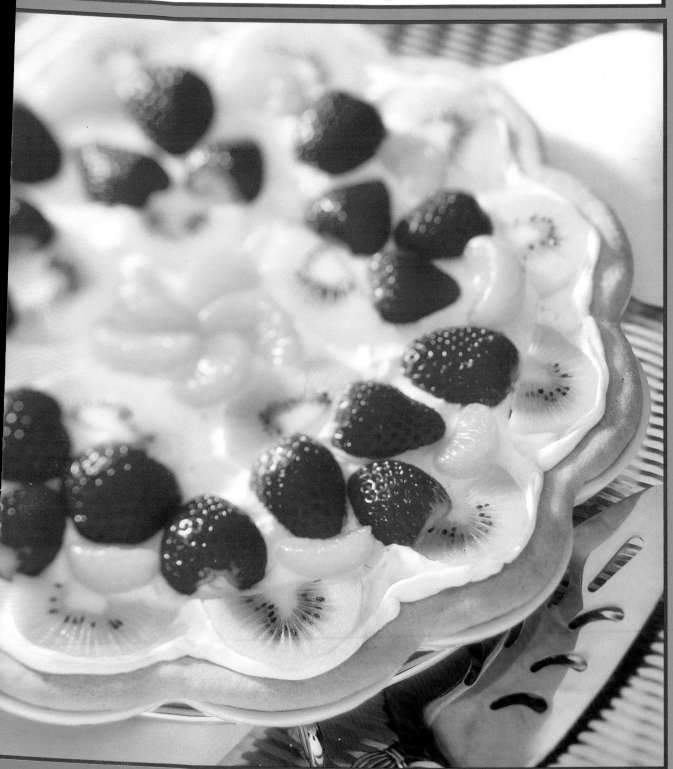

## Facts About Diabetes

Low-calorie, low-fat, low-cholesterol and low-sodium—buzzwords of the decade, and for a reason. People today are more aware than ever before of the roles diet and exercise play in maintaining a healthful lifestyle. For people with diabetes and their families, the positive impact good nutrition and physical activity have on well-being is very familiar.

Diabetes is a disease that affects the body's ability to use glucose as a source of fuel. When glucose is utilized improperly, it can build up in the bloodstream, creating higher-than-normal blood sugar levels. Left unchecked, elevated blood sugar levels may lead to the development of more serious long-term complications like blindness, heart disease and kidney disease.

Not all cases of diabetes are alike. In fact, the disease presents itself in two very distinct forms—Type I and Type II. Development of diabetes during childhood or adolescence is typical of Type I, or juvenile-onset, diabetes. These individuals are unable to make insulin, a hormone produced by the pancreas that moves glucose from the bloodstream into the body's cells, where the glucose is used as a source of fuel. Daily injections of insulin, coupled with a balanced meal plan, are the focus of treatment.

People who develop Type II diabetes, the more common form of the disease, are often over the age of 40 and are often overweight. These individuals produce insulin, but the amount produced may be insufficient to meet their needs; or their excess weight renders the hormone incapable of adequately performing its functions. Treatment typically includes balanced eating and exercise to reach and maintain a healthier weight. Some cases may require oral hypoglycemic agents or insulin injections prescribed by a doctor.

## Maximize Health, Minimize Complications

Diabetes increases one's risk of developing high blood pressure and high blood cholesterol levels. Over time, elevated blood sugar levels may progress to more serious complications, such as heart disease, kidney disease, stroke, hypertension, blindness, impotence or foot problems. In fact, research shows that individuals with diabetes are nineteen times more likely to develop kidney disease and four times more likely to suffer from heart disease or stroke than people who do not have diabetes. Regular appointments with your physician and registered dietitian or certified diabetes educator to fine-tune treatment strategies are good ways to help minimize complications. Strategies for treatment vary among individuals, yet overall goals remain the same: achieving and maintaining near-normal blood sugar levels by balancing food intake, physical activity and medications or insulin, if necessary; achieving optimal blood cholesterol levels; preventing complications and improving overall health through good nutrition.

## Balance Is the Key

Achieving optimal nutrition often requires lifestyle changes to balance the intake of nutrients. The United States Department of Agriculture and the United States Department of Health and Human Services developed the new 2000 Dietary Guidelines to simplify the basics of balanced eating, physical activity and safe food handling to help all individuals develop healthful eating plans. Because these recommendations are broad, work with your registered dietitian or certified diabetes educator and physician to personalize the guidelines to meet your specific needs.

## Aim for Fitness:

- Aim for a healthy weight.
- Be physically active each day.

### Build a Healthy Base:

- Let the Pyramid guide your food choices.
- Choose a variety of grains daily, especially whole grains.
- Choose a variety of fruits and vegetables daily.
- Keep food safe to eat.

### Choose Sensibly:

- Choose a diet that is low in saturated fat and cholesterol and moderate in total fat.
- Choose beverages and foods to moderate your intake of sugars.
- Choose and prepare foods with less salt.
- If you drink alcoholic beverages, do so in moderation.

**Use sugars in moderation.** In 1994, the American Diabetes Association lifted the absolute ban on sugar from the recommended dietary guidelines for people with diabetes. Under updated guidelines, you can, for example, exchange 1 tablespoon of sugar for a slice of bread because each is considered a starch exchange. The new guidelines for sugar intake are based on scientific studies that show that carbohydrate in the form of sugars does not raise blood glucose levels any more rapidly than other types of carbohydrate-containing food. What is more important is the total amount of carbohydrate eaten, not the source.

However, keep in mind that sweets and other foods high in sugar are usually high in calories and fat and contain few, if any, other nutrients, so the choice between an apple and a doughnut is still an easy one to make. Nobody, diabetic or not, should be eating foods filled with lots of sugar. But, when calculated into the nutritional analysis, a small amount of sugar can enhance a recipe and will not be harmful.

If you have any questions or concerns about incorporating sugar into your dietary meal plan, consult your certified diabetes educator, registered dietitian or physician for more information.

**Use salt and sodium in moderation.** Some people with diabetes may be more sensitive to sodium than others, making them more susceptible to high blood pressure. Minimize this risk by limiting sodium intake to no more than 2,400 mg a day (about 1 teaspoon of salt) and choosing single food items with less than 400 mg of sodium and entrées with less than 800 mg of sodium per serving.

## ABOUT THE RECIPES

The recipes in this cookbook were specifically developed for people with diabetes. All are based on the principals of sound nutrition as outlined by the dietary guidelines developed by the United States Department of Agriculture and the United States Department of Health and Human Services, making them perfect for the entire family.

Although the recipes are not intended as a medically therapeutic program, nor as a substitute for medically approved meal plans for individuals with diabetes, they contain amounts of calories, fat, cholesterol, sodium and carbohydrate that will fit easily into an individualized meal plan designed by your certified diabetes educator, registered dietitian or physician, and you.

The goal of this publication is to provide a variety of recipe choices for people with diabetes. Since diabetic meal plans can vary a great deal from one individual to another, not all recipes may be suitable for every person with diabetes. Therefore, choose wisely from the recipes in this book based on information provided by your certified diabetes educator, registered dietitian or physician, and your past experience.

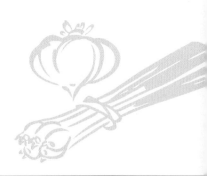

## Nutritional Analysis

The nutritional analysis that appears with each recipe was calculated by an independent nutritional consulting firm. Every effort has been made to check the accuracy of these numbers. However, because of a wide range of values in certain foods, all analyses that appear in this publication should be considered approximate.

• The analysis of each recipe includes all the ingredients that are listed in that recipe, except those labeled as "optional." Nutritional analysis is provided for the primary recipe only, not the recipe variation.

• If a range of amounts is offered for an ingredient (1 to 1¼ cups), the first amount given was used to calculate the nutritional information.

• If an ingredient is presented with an option ("1 cup hot cooked rice or noodles" for example), the first item listed was used to calculate the nutritional information.

• Foods shown in photographs on the same serving plate or offered as "serving suggestions" at the end of the recipe are not included in the recipe analysis unless they are listed in the ingredient list.

• In recipes calling for cooked rice or pasta or calling for rice or pasta to be cooked according to package directions, the analysis was based on preparation without salt and fat.

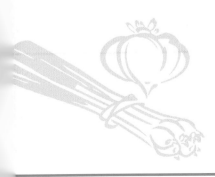

## Sugar Substitutes

Every recipe in this cookbook that uses a sugar substitute was developed using aspartame sweetener. Before making any of these recipes, check to see what kind of sugar substitute you are using (aspartame, acesulfame-k or saccharin). Look at the package carefully and use the amount necessary to equal the granulated sugar equivalent called for in each recipe. Follow the chart below for some general measurements. If you are using the product Diabeti Sweet, cooking and baking formula, this product is a one-to-one substitution for granulated sugar and no adjustments need to be made.

| Amount of Sugar Substitute Packets to Substitute for | | | |
| --- | --- | --- | --- |
| **Granulated Sugar** | **Aspartame** | **Acesulfame-K** | **Saccharin** |
| 2 teaspoons | 1 packet | 1 packet | ⅕ teaspoon |
| 1 tablespoon | 1½ packets | 1¼ packets | ⅓ teaspoon |
| ¼ cup | 6 packets | 3 packets | 3 packets |
| ⅓ cup | 8 packets | 4 packets | 4 packets |
| ½ cup | 12 packets | 6 packets | 6 packets |

# *Metric Conversion Chart*

## VOLUME MEASUREMENTS (dry)

⅛ teaspoon = 0.5 mL
¼ teaspoon = 1 mL
½ teaspoon = 2 mL
¾ teaspoon = 4 mL
1 teaspoon = 5 mL
1 tablespoon = 15 mL
2 tablespoons = 30 mL
¼ cup = 60 mL
⅓ cup = 75 mL
½ cup = 125 mL
⅔ cup = 150 mL
¾ cup = 175 mL
1 cup = 250 mL
2 cups = 1 pint = 500 mL
3 cups = 750 mL
4 cups = 1 quart = 1 L

## VOLUME MEASUREMENTS (fluid)

1 fluid ounce (2 tablespoons) = 30 mL
4 fluid ounces (½ cup) = 125 mL
8 fluid ounces (1 cup) = 250 mL
12 fluid ounces (1½ cups) = 375 mL
16 fluid ounces (2 cups) = 500 mL

## WEIGHTS (mass)

½ ounce = 15 g
1 ounce = 30 g
3 ounces = 90 g
4 ounces = 120 g
8 ounces = 225 g
10 ounces = 285 g
12 ounces = 360 g
16 ounces = 1 pound = 450 g

## DIMENSIONS

1/16 inch = 2 mm
⅛ inch = 3 mm
¼ inch = 6 mm
½ inch = 1.5 cm
¾ inch = 2 cm
1 inch = 2.5 cm

## OVEN TEMPERATURES

250°F = 120°C
275°F = 140°C
300°F = 150°C
325°F = 160°C
350°F = 180°C
375°F = 190°C
400°F = 200°C
425°F = 220°C
450°F = 230°C

## BAKING PAN SIZES

| Utensil | Size in Inches/Quarts | Metric Volume | Size in Centimeters |
|---|---|---|---|
| Baking or | 8×8×2 | 2 L | 20×20×5 |
| Cake Pan | 9×9×2 | 2.5 L | 23×23×5 |
| (square or | 12×8×2 | 3 L | 30×20×5 |
| rectangular) | 13×9×2 | 3.5 L | 33×23×5 |
| Loaf Pan | 8×4×3 | 1.5 L | 20×10×7 |
| | 9×5×3 | 2 L | 23×13×7 |
| Round Layer | 8×1½ | 1.2 L | 20×4 |
| Cake Pan | 9×1½ | 1.5 L | 23×4 |
| Pie Plate | 8×1¼ | 750 mL | 20×3 |
| | 9×1¼ | 1 L | 23×3 |
| Baking Dish | 1 quart | 1 L | — |
| or Casserole | 1½ quart | 1.5 L | — |
| | 2 quart | 2 L | — |

# Recipe Index

# Recipe Index

# Recipe Index

# Recipe Index

# *Recipe Index*

# Recipe Index